**Praise for *Hidden Mercy: AIDS, Catholics,
and the Untold Stories of Compassion in the Face of Fear***

"A superbly researched, beautifully written, and vividly presented portrait of an overlooked time in modern history. An important book about a key part of Catholic and American history that had to be written."
— James Martin, SJ, *New York Times* bestselling author of *Building a Bridge: How the Catholic Church and the LGBT Community Can Enter Into a Relationship of Respect, Compassion, and Sensitivity*

"With the precision and drive of an expert investigative journalist, the heart of a poet and the soul of a faithful, gay Catholic conflicted by his own spiritual home, his quest for answers about what the Church did, and did not do, in the mysterious and terrifying beginnings of AIDS in America unearths tragic yet beautiful stories of love and death that may have been lost without this magnificent and passionate documentary."
— Jeannie Gaffigan, author of *When Life Gives You Pears: The Healing Power of Family, Faith, and Funny People*

"Michael O'Loughlin sets his sights on an aspect of recent American history and culture too little examined. *Hidden Mercy* will cause discussion, argument, and maybe recommitment to an ideal of faith in action that can still play out in our day. And a good thing too."
— Gregory Maguire, *New York Times* bestselling author of *Wicked: The Life and Times of the Wicked Witch of the West*

"Michael J. O'Loughlin offers a moving personal history as well as a well written and reported account of the brave priests and nuns—queer and straight alike—that jeopardized their own career and standings with the church by merely treating LGBTQ Catholics with dignity during the height of the AIDS crisis."
— Michael Arceneaux, *New York Times* bestselling author of *I Can't Date Jesus: Love, Sex, Family, Race, and Other Reasons I've Put My Faith in Beyoncé* and *I Don't Want to Die Poor*

"O'Loughlin introduces us to so many unsung heroes of the AIDS crisis, and their lives vividly showcase the compassion and the cruelty that coexist in one community. A harrowing and deeply personal story."

—Molly Worthen, associate professor of history at the University of North Carolina at Chapel Hill, *New York Times* contributing opinion writer, and author of *Apostles of Reason: The Crisis of Authority in American Evangelicalism*

"*Hidden Mercy* isn't simply about institutional hypocrisy during the height of the AIDS years but also about the ongoing drive to build a more authentic, vibrant, and welcoming church from within, closer to the values of the Gospel. On top of all that it's compulsively readable, vigorous, and alive, full of searching, complicated, tough-minded, loving people."

—Paul Lisicky, author of *Later* and *The Narrow Door*

"Love—much like the power of community—really does stand at the center of *Hidden Mercy*. O'Loughlin never loses sight of that, and queer history is better because of it."

—Xorje Olivares, host of the podcast *Queer I Am, Lord*

"With care and curiosity, O'Loughlin weaves a compelling narrative that exists at the intersection of faith and sexuality. What follows is a story that is at times funny, surprising, and ultimately restores some of my own faith that people can and will show up for each other."

—Tobin Low, editor at *This American Life* and co-creator of the podcast *Nancy*

"Much has been written about how the Catholic Church failed us in the worst years of the AIDS pandemic. Michael O'Loughlin's deep reporting finds a much richer narrative."

—David France, author of *How to Survive a Plague*

HIDDEN MERCY

AIDS, CATHOLICS, AND THE UNTOLD STORIES OF
COMPASSION IN THE FACE OF FEAR

MICHAEL J. O'LOUGHLIN

BROADLEAF BOOKS
MINNEAPOLIS

HIDDEN MERCY
AIDS, Catholics, and the Untold Stories of Compassion in the Face of Fear

Cover image: Christopher Young—USA TODAY NETWORK
Cover design: Faceout Studios

Print ISBN: 978-1-5064-6770-2
eBook ISBN: 978-1-5064-6771-9

To Matt, with love and gratitude.

Contents

Evil crushes the lives of countless humans; there are few to intervene.

—Daniel Berrigan, SJ, To Dwell in Peace

Author's Note

The stories in this book originate from a range of sources, including organizational and personal archives, contemporaneous news reports, and more than one hundred interviews with people who lived and worked during the height of the HIV and AIDS crisis in the United States, roughly 1982 through 1996. The sources of any quotes taken from archival materials are provided in the endnotes. In most cases, they are drawn from my interviews and dialogue has been recreated based on the subject's recollection. Whenever possible, details have been checked against historical records. In a few instances, the sole source is one person's memory.

TIME WAS OF THE ESSENCE

New York

A Catholic nun from a small city in southern Illinois plopped herself down on a stool inside a dark New York City gay bar. It was 1987. Ronald Reagan was president. Madonna and Whitney Houston dominated the charts. *And the Band Played On* was a bestseller. But at that particular moment, Sister Carol Baltosiewich nursed her drink and glanced nervously around the bar. Small groups of men laughed. Some flirted; a few embraced. Sister Carol had so many questions. What were their stories? Where had they come from? How were they coping? For her, this was an entirely new world.

Born in 1943, Sister Carol was raised in a Polish-Catholic household outside Detroit. She later joined her religious order, the Hospital Sisters of Saint Francis, and graduated from nursing school, in 1971, before working in a handful of Midwestern hospitals. She was well educated and good at being a nurse. But none of that prepared her to be here, sipping a drink in a gay bar in New York City. She had no time to dwell on that, as she snapped back to reality when something caught her eye.

"What are they up to?" Sister Carol asked Will and Jim, a gay couple she had met a few weeks earlier. They were introducing her to their New York. Until then, her experience of the city had been limited to the convent where she was staying and the hospitals where she was volunteering. But Will and Jim's New York included gay bars. So from then on, with the couple as her guide, Sister Carol's New York would also include gay bars.

"Don't worry about that," Jim told her.

But Sister Carol was curious. She hadn't uprooted her life and moved into a convent in grimy Hell's Kitchen to have her questions go unanswered. Sister Carol was in New York *because* she had many questions. Complicated questions. Medical questions. But this question, wanting to know where the men were headed—that was simple. She wanted an answer.

"No, tell me," she protested. "Where is that guy going? And him, with all that leather?"

"OK, fine. We'll tell you," Jim said. "They're going to the baths."

"The baths?" Carol asked.

"Yeah, for sex. Anonymous sex," Carol remembers hearing, in a tone more matter-of-fact, she thought, than the words deserved.

"*Really?*" Carol asked.

She tried to hide her shock.

"Really," Jim said.

"Huh, OK," she replied.

Sister Carol still had much to learn. Was it really OK, like she had said? She wasn't sure. But that was enough question-and-answer for tonight.

A few weeks earlier, Sister Carol could never have imagined a scene like this. Back home in Belleville, Illinois, a sleepy city about twenty miles southeast of St. Louis, her life had become routine. She was a homecare nurse, visiting patients who were sick enough to need medical care but not so ill that they required hospitalization. She socialized with other sisters in her community. Her best friend was Sister Mary Ellen Rombach, a nurse and hospital chaplain who was a couple of decades older. They regularly ate dinner together. Over sandwiches, sometimes at a nearby Arby's, they recalled their days, griped about their patients, and chatted about the news.

When she was honest with herself, Sister Carol admitted that she was a little bored with homecare nursing. Previously, she had worked at a busy hospital in Wisconsin, attending to patients in the emergency department and the intensive care unit. But she had wanted out of the fast lane. That kind of work—dealing with literal matters of life and death, the constant buzzing of alarms, illness and organ failure and grieving families—burns people out. Sister Carol was no exception. She needed a break. So when she saw a listing for a home care nurse down in Illinois, she applied and got the job. She welcomed the relief a change of pace and scenery would offer. Sister Carol packed her stuff, trekked south to Belleville, and got right to work.

But one of her early patients dispelled the notion that the forty-four-year-old nurse nun was in for a break. The slower pace would be elusive. In fact, that patient would eventually lead Sister Carol to a gay bar a thousand miles away.

Scranton, Pennsylvania

A small plane landed in Scranton, Pennsylvania. On board was a soft-spoken Jesuit priest in his thirties named Father William Hart McNichols. Father McNichols had flown from New York City, where he had been living for the past few years. He had moved there from Denver in 1980 to study art at the Pratt Institute. Now well into the 1980s, he had seen the toll that HIV and AIDS were taking on young gay men, and he felt he had to do something to help. It wasn't just because as a priest, he was called to minister to the sick, though that was part of it. It was because he saw so much of himself reflected in those who were falling ill.

In the few years since he began his AIDS ministry, Father McNichols had become something of an expert on the subject, which led to this flight to Scranton. Father McNichols—known to many as "Father Bill"—was to be the Catholic representative at an interfaith HIV and AIDS ministry workshop. He was looking forward to sharing what he had learned through his work in Catholic hospitals in New York, the epicenter of the crisis. Plus the trip gave Father Bill something of a break from the city. Through his chaplaincy and informal AIDS ministry, he had run himself ragged.

What awaited him as he stepped off the plane sowed confusion. The organizer of the conference was there, along with a handful of reporters. Though he recognized that HIV and AIDS were very much in the news, Father Bill thought it a bit strange that members of the media were here to meet him at the airport. Perhaps he could answer whatever questions they had by talking about the unjust stigma facing people with AIDS, he thought to himself. Maybe he could even broach the controversial topic of religious leaders, including some of his own, perpetuating that stigma. After all, just the year before, the Vatican had released a letter condemning homosexuality, and as a result, gay and lesbian Catholics were being ejected from parishes across the country. Catholic bishops routinely fought against public health campaigns that promoted the use of condoms to fight HIV, and some even covered up the growing number of gay priests who had died from complications related to AIDS. The pain for gay and lesbian Catholics was raw. Perhaps there were valid reasons that the press might be stationed to meet the young Jesuit who was earning a reputation for challenging the views of church leaders.

"What do you think about the conference being canceled?" a reporter yelled, jolting Father Bill away from his thoughts and back to reality.

More confusion.

"The conference is canceled?" Father Bill asked one of the organizers. "Why?"

"Well, because of you," he sheepishly answered.

As they walked to the car, the organizer quietly explained what had happened. Though the conference was interfaith, most of the participants would be Catholic, given the demographics of that part of Pennsylvania. After the conference brochure was distributed, the organizers had received a call from the Catholic bishop's office. The bishop's representative said he was prohibiting Catholics from attending; because Father Bill was an outspoken advocate for gay and lesbian members of the church, he was not suitable to teach other Catholics. The organizers scrambled to make other plans, but with Catholics not allowed to attend, the numbers plummeted. The conference would have to be canceled.

Later, as Father Bill shared a meal with the organizers, he felt terrible. The hosts had paid for his flight and now their event had been scuttled. But he was also perplexed. He had no idea who would have worked behind the scenes to silence him. He didn't know anyone in Scranton, and he wasn't sure how his name had aroused suspicion here. Suddenly, he made the connection. Cardinal John O'Connor, the powerful, conservative archbishop of New York who had clashed repeatedly with the gay and lesbian community over his stance on gay rights, was previously the bishop of Scranton. Surely there was some connection. Father Bill apologized again and left to head back home.

Back in New York, he learned more of the story. Cardinal O'Connor, or likely someone from his office, had called contacts in Scranton and told them that Father Bill was not allowed to speak on behalf of the church. It was the 1980s. In the public square, gays demanded civil rights. Things were no different in the church. Gay and lesbian

Catholics wanted to be treated with dignity and respect. In response, some powerful Catholic leaders, including those in the Vatican and US bishops such as Cardinal O'Connor, cracked down. A culture war raged. The cancellation of the interfaith AIDS conference appeared to be yet another casualty.

Father Bill was hurt. He wasn't interested in scoring points or undermining the Catholic hierarchy. He just wanted people to listen to gay Catholics, to hear about their plight in the time of AIDS. But he didn't have time to dwell on the pain caused by the cancellation of his talk. He had buried too many friends. Too many young, gay men were still falling ill. Father Bill McNichols had work to do.

Chicago, Illinois, 2020

For as long as I can remember, I have been on a search. I am gay and I am Catholic. And I struggle continuously to reconcile those two parts of my identity. It feels ridiculous admitting this today, given the societal acceptance achieved by the LGBT community in recent years, but just typing the words "I am gay" fills my gut with a knot of anxiety. Not that long ago, I never would have been able to muster the courage to write such seemingly simple words, knowing they would be read by others. This anxiety doesn't make much sense, given my location as I write.

I'm sitting at an outdoor café in Boystown, the gay neighborhood I've chosen as my home. I'm surrounded by other people and I'm wearing a watch with a rainbow band. It's not exactly subtle. I originally bought the watchband to wear one June, Pride month, but I decided I liked the look and I keep it on year-round. That's not the only accessory I wear.

Around my neck, occasionally poking through the open buttons of my shirt, rests a silver chain. Affixed to it are a couple of medals emblazoned with images of saints. If someone were looking at me and noticed the watchband and the necklace, there would be no need for me to tell them I am gay and Catholic. They would know. But writing those words, or voicing them aloud, hasn't gotten much easier, even if I wear items that signify them silently. And that's the motivation for my search, a years-long attempt to unearth stories that help make these two indelible parts of my identity exist in peace. Or at least make me comfortable enough to say who I am without my cheeks warming and turning red.

Ask me to choose one over the other, gay or Catholic, and it would feel like asking someone to choose between having blonde hair or brown eyes. Hair dye or contacts could achieve either, I suppose, but deep down, there's really nothing you can do to change what is God-given. Plus, the choice doesn't make sense anyhow. That's how I've felt about my sexuality and my religious faith. I could leave the church, perhaps trying to find a more welcoming Christian community. They certainly exist. I toyed with that idea on more than one occasion, going so far as to set up a date to be received into a different Christian tradition. But I backed out before it ever happened. I also tried dating girls a couple of times, back in high school, but that wasn't fulfilling for anyone involved.

So I feel stuck. I am gay and I am Catholic, and I have to find a way to make this work. But this realization is easier said than done. Especially for someone like me, who perseverates on difficult questions, intent on finding satisfactory answers, not content to chalk up the problem as simply a great mystery.

My personal search for answers motivated some of my reporting when I first began working as a journalist. But it wasn't really a heavy lift. Given the battles over legalizing same-sex marriage when I began writing in 2009, I had the news on my side. I wasn't pitching stories about faith and sexuality that came out of left field, though I worried that editors and readers might catch on to why I so frequently wrote about LGBT issues. Polls that captured the attitudes of Catholics toward issues of sexual orientation? I covered them all. Comments from Catholic bishops opposing gay marriage? I tracked them down and wrote them up. I monitored social media, hiding behind my reporting while actively seeking out ideas on how others in my position made this all work. It all felt so new, so exciting. Had there ever been another time in history when empowered gay and lesbian people of faith asserted their rights and won? I didn't think so.

But a few years of this kind of writing hadn't resulted in too much progress for me personally. It was all too sterile. Polls and statements didn't prompt the kind of meaningful conversation I craved, so I decided to look deeper. In 2013, I pitched a story about LGBT resources on Catholic university campuses. Did college-age Catholics now demand more respect than when I was a student? Reporting that story involved a return to Saint Anselm College in New Hampshire to see firsthand the changes taking place in the ten years since I had enrolled as a freshman.

Back then, in 2003, it felt like an implicit "don't ask, don't tell" policy was in effect when it came to gay and lesbian students. There were no LGBT student groups on campus, and sometimes it seemed as if there weren't any other gay students, period. But we eventually found each other. We might roll our eyes when recounting a passing comment against homosexuality made by a professor, but we would also rejoice during those rare moments when we felt affirmed, publicly and without shame. Like the time when the president of the college, a Benedictine monk named Father Jonathan DeFelice, preached at a Mass during family weekend, stating unequivocally that gay students and their families were as welcome on campus as anyone else. A small line that I am sure most attendees have long since forgotten, but one that meant the world to me.

In many ways the college just didn't really think about gay or lesbian students, a fact that sometimes provided us what some others might consider special treatment. Dorms were separated by gender. Boys lived with other boys and girls with other girls. The rules prohibited comingling after a certain hour. As for hosting overnight guests of the opposite sex, don't even think about it. Resident assistants patrolled the hallways at night, listened for sounds of unwelcome visitors, kicked them out, and wrote up warnings. But what if a semi-closeted sophomore who lived in a single room in one of the all-boys' dorms wished to host a male friend for the night? What if that friend started appearing with some regularity? Well, no one raised an eyebrow to me about that. It was a nice perk, but surely LGBT students deserved more.

Through my reporting for the story, I learned that a decade after my undergraduate experience, some Catholic schools now offered many more LGBT resources. Some had entire offices, staffs, and programs devoted exclusively to this group of students, though those schools admittedly seemed to be the exception. Others offered nothing at all and seemed, in fact, to punish students who dared to raise the topic. My college, I discovered, was somewhere in the middle. In the years after I graduated, some students had asked to create an LGBT student group. The school agreed to the request but laid out some conditions, including that the new organization be housed in campus ministry, not student activities. That structure ensured that no lines would be crossed when it came to challenging the church's teaching against homosexuality.

When my story was published, mostly positive feedback arrived in my inbox. Other LGBT people who attended Catholic colleges and universities were eager to tell me about their experiences. Many readers assumed I was gay, even if I didn't say so explicitly in the report. These emails served as a nudge, urging me to keep searching for answers.

Shortly after, in June 2013, news events involving the intersection of faith and sexuality showed no signs of slowing. Later that summer, the newly installed Pope Francis responded to a journalist's question about gay priests by asking, "Who am I to judge?" That simple answer from the still relatively unknown pope set off a flurry of hopeful commentary from gay Catholics, myself included. Only my commentary required something of an asterisk. I still wasn't out—at least not publicly. That reality didn't stop me from writing an essay about how the pope's comments provided hope to LGBT Catholics. The evidence I supplied was based on my interviews with *those* kinds of Catholics; I didn't let my own experience drive the essay. It was a piece that would make some editors scream—a personal reflection, but one exclusively highlighting other people. It would have been more powerful coming from someone with enough courage to admit the real reason he found the pope's words so moving was because they spoke directly to him.

My essay was apparently insightful enough, however, that the influential blogger Andrew Sullivan, another gay Catholic, excerpted the piece. At first, I was elated, grateful for the boost. But as I read through the post and reached the section quoting my work, I panicked. There I was, identified as a "gay Catholic." Yikes. Though I was out to some friends, family, and colleagues, I worked for a Catholic organization. I worried about my job. What would people in my professional circle think?

A few days went by. Nothing bad happened. Several people told me that they liked my essay, but that was it. The closet I had constructed for myself was made of crystal-clear glass, it seemed, so no one appeared all that shocked by my being labeled a "gay Catholic." Plus, most people simply didn't care. The experience proved to be a relief, leaving me more confident and willing to take more risks.

I began talking openly with friends, coworkers, and other "professional Catholics" about my own experiences. I decided to write more personally, though I still held back a bit, never overtly describing myself as gay. In March 2014, I appeared on MSNBC to talk about a piece I had written for the LGBT magazine *The Advocate*. I argued it was unfair to ban gay groups from Saint Patrick's Day parades in Boston and New York and highlighted how even some church leaders now seemed to agree.

When the interview finished, a producer said through an earpiece that he thought I did well. He told me to enjoy a Guinness that afternoon.

The following month, in April 2014, I wrote an essay in *Foreign Policy* urging the pope to speak out against the criminalization of homosexuality around the globe. Later that spring, I even accepted an invitation to join a working group at the State Department, serving as a Catholic representative to talk about global faith and sexuality. Through this work, I received an invitation to the United States Naval Observatory, the vice president's home, where I sipped white wine around the pool with other gay leaders. I stood in line for a photo with then Vice President Joe Biden and Dr. Jill Biden. When it was finally my turn, I used my few seconds with the nation's first Catholic vice president to thank him for his courage in supporting marriage equality. He smiled. I smiled. The camera clicked. And I went on my way.

Professionally, things continued like this for the next few years. The *Boston Globe* hired me to cover US Catholicism, something of a dream job, writing for the newspaper I had read growing up in Massachusetts. I visited Cincinnati to report a feature about a new morality clause that effectively banned gay teachers in Catholic schools. In Los Angeles, I interviewed transgender Catholics about their hopes for the church. I traveled to Rome to cover a global meeting of bishops about family issues, where I somehow mustered up the courage to ask influential cardinals how they planned to make the church more welcoming to gay Catholics and their families. In short, I grew more comfortable asking questions about these issues, seeking answers for both my readers and myself as I tried to make life as a gay Catholic work for me. Yet I still felt like I couldn't be honest with people about my personal life. I was having trouble integrating that side of myself with my faith. I needed insight from people with more experience, people who had lived through similar struggles. But who?

Then my prayers seemed to be answered.

Over dinner one evening, in 2015, a friend told me a story that would change the course of my life for the next several years.

My friend, a couple of decades older than me, told me that when he was a young priest, gay Catholics had faced fierce backlash from church authorities cracking down on unorthodoxy, just as HIV and AIDS upended their lives. These twin crises created a pressure cooker. My friend ministered to some of these struggling Catholics. Their stories stuck with him even decades later. He shared a few with me. I was hooked.

"There's a lot there," he told me. He encouraged me to learn more of this history, thinking it might make my own search for integration more fruitful.

After this conversation, I was intent on learning more about the interactions between LGBT Catholics and church leaders during the height of the AIDS crisis in the United States. I didn't know much of this history at all. Various facts from the 1980s lived inside my head, but they were like isolated stars, never forming a constellation that could illuminate that time.

Like many gay Catholics in their early thirties, perhaps, I knew on some level that tension existed between the church and gay activists in the 1980s. I even understood that much of the frustration revolved around the use of condoms in fighting the spread of HIV. But a huge gap existed in my understanding of my own community. I eventually would come to learn why.

History about LGBT people often isn't passed on from generation to generation. It's not recounted around the dinner table and hasn't been taught widely in public schools. Priests tend not to highlight it from the pulpit. Of the thousands of Catholic saints, not a single one is identified as gay or lesbian. Intergenerational friendships are also all too rare in the gay community. If these were more common, perhaps I would have known more of this history. My history.

That realization gave me an idea.

Rather than lament that others had not taught me this important history, I decided to take responsibility for my own education. Over the next few years, I used the skills I acquired as a reporter to locate people whose stories might help me find answers. I reached out with emails and phone calls to introduce myself. I offered a bit of my story and hoped they would be willing to share theirs. Time was of the essence. The people I talked to were in their sixties and seventies. On many occasions, after asking for more details about a particular story, they would say something like, "Oh, you would have loved talking to so and so, but they died a few years ago." These stories risked being lost to history. I had my work cut out for me.

I sorted through dusty archives in quiet libraries. I cold-called people who had been involved in AIDS work. I asked for interviews. I talked to a doctor who treated people with AIDS from the earliest days of the crisis, first in San Francisco and later in Boston. He also happens to be a Jesuit priest, named Father Jon Fuller, who introduced me to several members of the organization he once ran, the National Catholic AIDS Network. I interviewed activists from the AIDS Coalition to Unleash Power, or ACT UP. They had taken on Wall Street, drug companies, the Reagan administration, and the Catholic Church. I spent time in the homes and workplaces of gay Catholics who remember vividly the horror of the earliest days of AIDS—even if they hadn't talked about the trauma in decades. Many of them told me about the anger they felt, and sometimes still feel, when thinking about how their church opted to bruise and batter their souls rather than offer a balm for their wounds. Somehow, through it all, many of them kept their faith. I took notes, asked questions, thumbed through their scrapbooks.

Through these meetings and phone calls, I learned a history that had previously been denied to me, one that could have helped me understand that my personal struggle was less unique than it sometimes felt. Later, I would come to learn that this feeling of isolation isn't unusual for young

LGBT people, especially those of us trying to find a home in what can often feel like an unwelcoming religious tradition.

What made a priest or a nun willing to jeopardize their own ministry and reputation and stand with LGBT Catholics? I asked some who had done just that. What was it like to feel rejected by your church because of your sexual orientation—and what made some LGBT people stay faithful anyway? I found gay Catholics who had protested the church's teaching on homosexuality in the 1980s and I asked them. And how did people cope as they watched partners and friends die from a disease that society didn't care about, only to be turned away by their church when they most needed spiritual support? I contacted long-term survivors who are facing the challenges of aging with HIV, without networks of long-time friends who might intimately understand their struggles, because so many of them had died from AIDS decades earlier.

———

Back at the Boystown café, reflecting on the stories I've learned during this search, I recall with gratitude the many people whose lives have helped make me slightly more comfortable writing that simple sentence: I am gay and I am Catholic. The fact that I can write that at all is a testament to the graciousness so many others have shown in sharing their memories with me. I know there are many more stories I have yet to learn. There are omissions in this book. Some are obvious and I will later regret not having included them, and some I won't know anything about until readers contact me to reveal something personal from their lives. Many other stories have simply been lost to time, names and memories long forgotten.

But I hope I do justice to the stories of Sister Carol and Father Bill and the many others who entrusted me with some of their most private moments. It might go without saying, but each person in this book is unique. Some are straight, some are gay. Some don't say either way. Some were born and raised Catholic and never left the church, and some protested against it and eventually exited when they saw it failing to live up to its own ideals. Some seemed to thrive during the chaos of the AIDS crisis. Others broke down crying when they recounted friends and loved ones whose deaths feel as fresh as they did back then. Between 1980 and 1996, more than 581,000 Americans were diagnosed with AIDS, mostly gay men. More than 362,000 of them died, after enduring the shame and stigma that so often accompanied their diagnosis and lacking even the comfort of knowing that the wider society was fighting a cure. Some of those lost lives are recalled here as well, relying on memories to help remember the dead. Though each story takes different twists and turns, many of the people I interviewed for this book have at least one thing in common. They were willing to offer insights about a time in history filled with pain, grief, hope, anger, love, and loss, in an effort to keep this history alive and introduce it to others so that we might feel less alone.

2

"THROUGH THEIR OWN FAULT"

Unearthing stories that I hoped would help me figure out life as a gay Catholic began with a literal search: an effort to find a piece of architectural history that I was told is essential to see firsthand if I wanted to understand the Catholic Church's role in responding to AIDS.

My colleague Anna Marchese and I tried to locate somebody, anybody, who would give us a tour of a certain church in Greenwich Village. The parish, Saint Veronica's, was established in the late 1800s to serve Irish dockworkers who needed a place to pray, socialize, and send their kids to school. But more than a century later, with the neighborhood looking nothing like it had during the parish's heyday, when affordable row houses were filled with young families, the church was slated to close. Gaining access to the building before the final Mass in a couple of days was proving difficult. But we finally found a former parishioner and local historian who agreed to show us around.

On a steamy July morning, I left my hotel and took the train downtown for a quick breakfast before Anna and I headed to Saint Veronica's. All I knew about Saint Veronica's was its location in a neighborhood that was synonymous with New York's gay culture and that the parish had a connection to AIDS. If the archdiocese closed the parish, I learned, New Yorkers would be cut off from the city's first AIDS memorial. This was striking, because AIDS memorials were relatively rare, a shocking level of disregard given the number of deaths attributed to HIV and AIDS and the fact that it's still an ongoing crisis. Given the deep divisions between the church and the gay community, it surprised me that one of the nation's first AIDS memorials was housed inside a Catholic parish. We wanted to see it before it was too late.

The facade of Saint Veronica's is a striking burgundy brick, with two terra-cotta–topped steeples rising above the surrounding rowhouses. Inside, the church was empty. The sanctuary had been restored a few years earlier, but the building still bore unmistakable signs of another era: high ceilings cut with elaborate stained glass, columns of faux brown marble, bronzed candle stands, and a high altar separated by a white marble rail. The interior was brighter than many churches, with light pouring in through a huge oculus cut into the ceiling, a reminder of the novelty of electricity when the church was constructed. Some of the gas jets once used to illuminate lanterns remained protruding from the walls.

Part of the church's history, we learned, included a parish-wide response to the HIV crisis. In 1985, Cardinal O'Connor granted Mother Teresa's request for a piece of archdiocesan property to open an AIDS hospice. The cardinal offered the rectory at Saint Veronica's, moving the priests residing there to a nearby house. On Christmas Eve, Mayor Ed Koch and Cardinal O'Connor joined Mother Teresa, who sported a pair of aviator sunglasses on account of recent cataract surgery, to open the facility. She described it as a guest house for people with AIDS, and the first residents were prisoners who had been granted medical furlough by the governor at her request.

Around the same time, gay activists in the neighborhood organized candlelight vigils to remember people who had died from AIDS and to raise awareness about the ongoing struggle. Some of the vigils weaved through Greenwich Village, passing by Saint Veronica's. A new pastor arrived in 1990, at which point more than 120,000 Americans had died from AIDS, and he thought Saint Veronica's should do more to respond to the crisis. He reached out to local gay leaders but encountered some initial skepticism. Just a year earlier, activists had targeted the Catholic Church in a major demonstration at Saint Patrick's Cathedral. Feelings were still raw. But after a few meetings, the pastor and activists created a plan for the church to host interfaith AIDS prayer services. By the summer of 1992, an idea to place an AIDS memorial inside the church had been realized.

Our guide told us the memorial was upstairs in the lower choir loft. When we entered the church, we noticed a plaque dedicated to members of the parish who had died during World War II, affixed to a spot that was visible to everyone who assembled for Sunday Mass. That the AIDS memorial was located so far away, high in the choir loft, seemed off to me. I shrugged my shoulders, and we climbed the stairs. Sure enough, there in front of the first pew was the Saint Veronica's AIDS Memorial, a series of small, bronze-colored plaques glued to a dark brown wooden rail. "In memory of all the people we have loved and lost to AIDS," read one. "To live in the hearts of those we leave behind is to never die." Situated on either side were hundreds of names, mostly of young men, who had died from AIDS.

Families and friends bought individual plaques to memorialize their loved ones inside the church. It wasn't uncommon, especially in the early 1990s, to see middle-aged women sitting in the choir loft alone, quietly crying, presumably the mothers of the young men who had died. It was quite moving, heartbreaking even, our guide told us. I could tell she was sincere in her description of how the site spoke to her and how it motivated her fight to preserve the building.

And yet, as I sat looking at the memorial, at the small plaques listing name after name, I felt a mix of emotions. Thinking of those young men, living in New York with their whole lives ahead of them, only to succumb to a new disease while being shunned by society, caused a physical reaction. My shoulders tensed, and I clenched my jaw. The injustice of it all weighed on me. The memorial's obscurity felt wrong. Was this really the best the church could do to honor young gay men killed by AIDS? I appreciated that the installation at Saint Veronica's was at least an attempt to remember people whose lives had been cut short. But its location felt like good intentions had been overshadowed by a sense of shame, a hint of something blameworthy in how these men died—that perhaps there was something wrong with being gay.

———

By the time I visited Saint Veronica's, I had learned about the stigma and shame that too often accompanies a diagnosis of HIV or a death caused by AIDS. For people like me who don't remember the crisis firsthand, it can feel impossible to comprehend how seemingly every sector of society responded to AIDS with callous indifference or even outright contempt.

Throughout the 1960s and '70s, gay and lesbian Americans were no longer willing to live in the shadows. For too long, society's gatekeepers had prevented them from being open about their sexuality, or from building lives with the people they loved, simply because they happened to be of the same sex. A series of sometimes violent protests in 1969, attributed to a riot against police brutality, at a New York gay bar called the Stonewall Inn, advanced the cause of gay rights. By the late 1970s, communities of LGBT people had grown even more assertive. There was a sense they were winning, that the public would come around to their side. Because, they argued, liberation for gay and lesbian people would advance the cause of justice for all Americans.

But that confidence came at a cost, in the form of an equally vocal backlash. It's easy to lay the blame solely at the feet of religious conservatives, who certainly helped perpetuate the idea that homosexuality was a sin. But even non-religious political leaders, elite journalists, and medical professionals refused to accept gay people. There was just something not quite right about people who would choose to live "that way." When gays were relegated to the margins, it was easy to ignore them. When they began holding rallies and parades, condemning this "alternative lifestyle" became fashionable in some circles. The push and pull continued for years, with gays demanding equal rights and conservatives digging in their heels.

Then AIDS hit, seeming to herald just what the opponents of gay liberation had been warning about: *that* kind of lifestyle couldn't go unpunished for long.

At first, there was just a trickle of confirmed cases. Nearly all of them were confined to gay men living in large, coastal urban centers. The media was hesitant to go near the story, since homosexuality was not appropriate to cover in a family newspaper. Plus, even open-minded scientists weren't yet sure what this was. Was it cancer? But a cancer that seemingly affected only a small subset of the population? That didn't make sense. Maybe it was simply a cluster of illness that would burn out on its own.

Eventually answers would arrive. First called "gay-related immune deficiency" or GRID, the disease by 1982 came to be called the acquired immunodeficiency syndrome, or AIDS, and by 1984, it was discovered that AIDS was spread by HIV, the human immunodeficiency virus. In effect, "acquired immunodeficiency" meant that the illness was characterized by a breakdown of the body's natural ability to fight infection. A person with a healthy immune system has anywhere between 500 and 1,600 infection-fighting T-cells per cubic millimeter of blood. Over time, HIV destroys these T-cells, causing their numbers to decline. If an HIV-positive person's T-cells drop below 200, or if the individual develops opportunistic infections, that person progresses from being HIV-positive to having AIDS. In a person with a healthy immune system, infections such as pneumonia and even certain kinds of cancers can pose minimal risk. For people with AIDS, in the early days of the crisis, they were almost always deadly.

Scientific research showed the virus was present in blood and semen and therefore required the exchange of bodily fluids in order to spread. Despite the fact that this was a more limited mode of transmission than many other viruses, the lack of widespread knowledge about HIV in the early days, combined with its deadly nature, sparked deep fear. And as it so often does, fear led to hate.

The case numbers were dramatic. By the end of 1981, 159 cases of AIDS were reported in the entire United States. Just six years later, when Sister Carol arrived in New York, more than 50,000 Americans were diagnosed with AIDS and nearly 41,000 had already died from the disease. The number of AIDS deaths per year finally began to decline in 1996, but not before 362,000 Americans had died. Put another way, more people than the entire population of Pittsburgh perished over a fifteen-year period.

But the numbers alone fail to tell the whole story.

———

Early on, the group most affected by HIV and AIDS was composed of gay men. A relatively small community bore the brunt of the disease, one that already felt besieged from all sides. The people I interviewed painted vivid pictures of the trauma they experienced during this time. One man told me about the first friends he made when he moved to San Francisco in the 1980s: two drag queens who took him under their wings. Both would die from AIDS just a few years later. Then he lost most of his other friends over the next few years. A Catholic nun who worked in a hospital with a large patient population of gay men with AIDS recalled entire apartment buildings being emptied out over the course of just a few months, each resident getting sick and then dying from this horrible disease a few weeks later.

On top of the physical suffering was layered an uncaring and at times overtly hostile public. Around the time that Sister Carol and Sister Mary Ellen began exploring HIV and AIDS ministry, for example, a national poll found that a quarter of Americans believed "AIDS is a punishment God has given homosexuals for the way they live." A third of Americans believed sex between gay people should be illegal. And those views weren't confined to small cities and towns like Belleville. Even in New York, stigma was rampant. Including among Catholics.

A group of neighbors in New York City's Upper West Side, for example, became irate in the summer of 1985 when the archdiocese announced plans to open a shelter for people with AIDS, its first venture into HIV and AIDS care. The Missionaries of Charity, Mother Teresa's nuns, agreed to staff the shelter. The archdiocese chose a piece of property that would be converted, attached to Holy Name of Jesus Church on Ninety-Sixth Street The location, a former convent located near the church and parish school, was ideal because it was not far from Saint Clare's, a Catholic hospital with a planned unit dedicated to HIV and AIDS.

Except the neighbors weren't having any of it.

When the church announced the news in the Sunday bulletin, parishioners mobilized in opposition. In just a few days, several hundred had signed a petition. They were "shocked" that a former convent would be used to house people with AIDS. If the plans went forward, they warned, they would keep their kids home from the parish school. That meant five hundred empty desks—and unpaid tuition bills.

"Right now, no one knows the whole cause [of the disease]," one parent told a reporter, articulating the fear that surrounded the disease. "It could be discovered [that] spit could transfer AIDS. We're not going to take that chance."

The parish hosted a homeless shelter in its basement, which some parishioners thought was enough social action. AIDS? That was going too far. The pastor was furious with his flock, preaching to them at weekend Masses, "Wherever there is a victim of AIDS, Jesus Christ is there." Nonetheless, the archdiocese canceled the plans in August 1985, though it eventually found another location in Greenwich Village—at Saint Veronica's—and this time it did not alert the neighbors to the plans in advance.

The homophobia that fueled petition drives and boycotts was pervasive and could appear in the most mundane of places.

Riding the subway was normally uneventful for another Catholic nun active in AIDS ministry, Sister Pascal Conforti. She boarded the train near her convent in the Bronx and made her way to Fiftieth Street in Hell's Kitchen. From there, she walked to Saint Clare's Hospital, where Sister Carol volunteered. Normally the journey went off without a hitch. But on this particular morning, Sister Pascal noticed a woman looking at her. She was middle aged and dressed like she was on her way to work. When the train stalled for a bit, just shy of the stop, the woman introduced herself. She was a member of her parish rosary society. A good Catholic.

"Where are you going?" she asked Sister Pascal.

"I'm going to Saint Clare's," she explained, naming the nearby hospital where she was a chaplain on the AIDS ward.

"Oh," the woman said, with a tone that let Sister Pascal know more words were coming. "That's the place."

Sister Pascal raised an eyebrow.

"That's where all those people who have AIDS go," she continued. There was a pause. "*I* don't have to worry about that."

Against her better judgment, Sister Pascal took the bait. She didn't put up with ignorance of any kind. As one of her colleagues at the hospital described her, she was simultaneously "a living saint" and "one badass nun."

"And why is that?"

"Well, I never do anything wrong."

The implication was clear: Only people who "did things wrong" ended up dying in an AIDS ward. This wasn't the first time Sister Pascal had encountered Catholics who looked at her AIDS work with suspicion. One time, a man asked her why she "wasted time with people who were ill through their own fault."

Those judgmental words, evocative of what she had just heard from the woman on the train, were so distant from the love she saw in the hospital. She had counseled hundreds of men with AIDS, mostly poor and gay, including prisoners and sex workers. She listened to their stories and accompanied them through their final days. She daily stood in awe of their deep spirituality and selfless love.

She thought of Henry, who had been diagnosed with HIV, and his partner, Bernie, who cared for him. When Henry took a turn for the worse and developed AIDS, he was admitted to Saint Clare's. He was dying. When it became clear the end was near, a priest was summoned. He prayed over Henry, rubbed oil on his forehead, and blessed him. But Bernie was upset. The love of his life was dying. They were both too young to be dealing with this. Bernie wasn't Christian, but he turned to Sister Pascal for comfort. Part of her job, she understood, was to minister to people in pain. She thought about the ritual they had just witnessed, one that seemed to move Bernie even if he didn't fully grasp the theology behind it. He asked what it all meant.

"The bottom line is one lifetime perhaps isn't enough to hold the love of the human heart," Sister Pascal told Bernie. "There's some way in which love continues. The spirit continues in mysterious ways." Bernie was moved by Sister Pascal's image, comforted for the time being.

Sister Pascal was sick of well-meaning people saying in response to stories about her AIDS work that it was important to "love the sinner and hate the sin." It was arrogant, and she didn't want to hear it. She said as much to the woman on the train before leaving for her walk to the hospital.

There was a job to do. People were sick and in need of care. Sister Pascal made her case and went on her way to visit patients.

The kind of prejudice voiced by the woman on the subway was present in nearly every facet of society. The White House press corps laughed in 1982 when a reporter asked a question about AIDS, referring to the epidemic's seriousness by calling it a "gay plague." President Reagan's spokesman responded with a homophobic joke: "I don't have it; do you?" The reporters laughed again as the banter continued. As for the president himself, he didn't give a major speech about AIDS until 1987, six years into the crisis, when the "gay plague" moniker had become common, further stigmatizing a beleaguered community. And in the Catholic Church, mainstream bishops fought vigorously against gay rights and some fringe figures bought into the fatal theology that presented AIDS as a punishment from God. But most people simply seemed to ignore the problem altogether.

Which is what makes Father Bill and Sister Carol so extraordinary.

3

HOSPITAL SISTERS

The first time Sister Carol and I speak is in July 2016. On that call, she seems a little surprised that I have contacted her. Her voice is somewhat diminutive, kind if not effusively warm. There's a clicking in the background. Carol says it's her oxygen tank. I tell her she is my first phone interview for what I hope will become a book about the Catholic Church's response to the early days of the HIV and AIDS crisis.

"Huh," Sister Carol says, before pausing for a moment. "Why?"

It's a seemingly simple and expected question: "Why?" But it's one that I've steeled myself for, dreading that it will be asked but knowing that it deserves an answer. If a stranger calls out of the blue and asks you to share a chapter of your life that you had long ago packed away, in both literal and figurative boxes, it's natural to ask, "Why?"

But as a reporter, I've learned it's best not to reveal too much about my own life to people I interview. Especially priests and nuns. I often evade questions that might require disclosing something personal, either by offering vague answers or by swiftly moving on to a new topic. It's still difficult to talk about myself, my own sexual orientation, especially with other Catholics. But in this instance, I don't want Sister Carol to sense something is off and thus not feel comfortable opening up with me. I perceive there is a great story here and that she could offer insight that could help other people. Even in the few minutes that we've been talking, I've gotten the sense that she would want a clear answer before going much further. I take a deep breath and answer her question.

"Why? Well, I'm gay. I'm Catholic," I say. "And I've been wrestling with those two parts of myself for a long time."

"Oh," Sister Carol says matter-of-factly, without a hint of judgment. "OK."

OK. Her answer is simultaneously affirming and, if I'm being honest, a bit of letdown. It seems she holds no animosity toward gay people. This is hardly surprising, given her decade of work in AIDS care. But it's also somehow deflating, because in my head I've created a narrative that I need to be on the defensive when outing myself to priests and nuns. Even though I've had almost nothing but positive experiences in these situations, there's something about meeting a church leader for the first time that makes me want to hide my true identity. All that adrenaline builds up, and Carol immediately disarms me with her "OK."

My answer seems good enough for her, and our conversation continues. I explain that her story had been one of the first I encountered in an AIDS archive I was exploring at home in Chicago. I'm eager to hear more.

"Got it," she responds. "Well, here's my story."

Sister Carol and I talk for the next two hours. I record the interview on my phone, and my hands cramp from trying to type every word she speaks. Her story fascinates me. Her candor is refreshing and her sense of moral clarity inspiring. When we finish the interview, I thank her, but I apologize because I don't yet know how the material will be used. A book, I hope. Maybe an article.

"Anyway," I say. "Let's stay in touch."

"Sounds good," she says.

Another year goes by before Sister Carol and I reconnect. In the meantime, I continue researching. When a publisher accepts a pitch for a story about the church's response to AIDS, I ask Carol if I can visit Belleville to conduct a proper interview, hoping it will be worthwhile to meet in person. She says yes and offers to contact old friends who can provide more details about their time working in AIDS ministry. Plus, she tells me, I'll be able to see the fruits of her labor: a resource center for people with HIV and AIDS that is still in operation.

———

On a frigid February morning in 2018, my iPhone alarm blares at five a.m., an ungodly hour for me. I rub the sleep out of my eyes, hop in the shower, and dress in layers. The night before, anticipating the early start, I packed my things. Change of clothes. Toothbrush. Audio recorder and notebook. With my bag slung over my shoulder, I head to Union Station for the five-hour train ride from Chicago to St. Louis. As the train nears Springfield, I start getting nervous. Gray skies and an endless expanse of fallow fields provide no immediate distraction.

"What am I doing?" I think.

As the train pulls into the station, I tell myself there's no turning back. Sister Carol is expecting me, and it would be rude to cancel. I jump in a rental car, check in at the hotel, and snap a selfie in front of the Gateway Arch, something to distract myself from my growing anxiety. Will she and I have enough to talk about? Was I crazy for coming all the way down here? I snap out of the doom spiral as I check my watch. I have to hit the road to make it across the Mississippi River to Belleville in time for our meeting.

When I finally arrive at Sister Carol's home, in a modest apartment complex off a busy, multi-lane road, a small dog barks loudly after I ring the doorbell.

"Give me a minute," Carol calls out.

I wait on the stoop, staring down at a concrete statue of Saint Francis of Assisi. Sister Carol apologizes as she opens the door. I shove my hands in my pockets. Plastic oxygen tubing is inserted under her nose and runs across the length of the floor into a tank nestled atop a plush chair. She welcomes me inside and shoos the dog into a bedroom. She tells me she has a couple good hours left before she'll get tired, so we had better get to work.

Sister Carol fills me in about her upbringing in Detroit and her decision to become a Catholic nun and go into nursing. She starts to explain how she became involved in AIDS care but stops suddenly when she has an idea.

"Hang tight while I get some photo albums," she tells me.

I save the audio file and glance down at my watch. It's getting dark and I have to drive back to St. Louis. Carol and I had planned to meet again in the morning, so I decide I'll ask if we can wait to look through the albums. Plus, I'm tired and hungry. This can all wait.

But when Carol returns, something has changed in her demeanor. It appears the albums have awakened vivid memories. Gone is the brisk pace in the telling of her war stories. She suddenly remembers illuminating details she had previously overlooked.

Names come back. She laughs, recalling a particularly memorable dinner with a group of gay men who had befriended her. She flips through one album, filled with photos of men in their twenties and thirties, dressed casually in that unmistakable 1980s style. In one, two gay men are snuggled up next to each other, kept warm in red and white hooded sweatshirts. In another, Sister Carol sits with a group of five gay men around a bar table, empty cans of Miller Lite piling up. She looks happy in the photos, a wide smile plastered across her face. She points to one picture, her wrinkled hand showing how she has aged since the photos were taken. Sadness creeps into her voice.

"He died," she says, indicating a portrait of one young man, his name written in perfect Catholic-school penmanship below. "Him too. Oh, this was taken right before he got sick. And then he died."

She looks down for what feels like several minutes.

"So many of them," she says quietly, "all gone."

Sister Carol worked with people with AIDS for about a decade. She became a leading advocate in Illinois for expanded HIV testing, funding for AIDS care, and anti-stigma education. She would be featured in local news reports about HIV and AIDS and named to a state commission to help disperse much-needed funding in a fair and equitable manner. But that would all come later. To reach that point, Sister Carol would first have to learn the ins and outs of caring for people in their homes, listening to their needs, and using her nursing skills to get the job done. And as a Catholic nun who had grown up in conservative Midwestern enclaves, she would have to confront how her church's teachings about homosexuality influenced her own work and views.

———

Outside Chicago, much of Illinois is largely rural. The city of Belleville may be a relatively short drive from St. Louis, but it's a decidedly low-key community. A single strip of businesses constitutes the center of town, while small houses and budget hotels dot the landscape alongside the highway. Head out a little farther from Belleville and fields spread as far as the eye can see.

Sister Carol's AIDS ministry began there, unwittingly, in 1984. She had just turned forty and settled into her new job, leaving behind the frenetic pace of the ER for homecare nursing. One of her first assignments took her to a farmhouse about an hour from home, where a woman needed help recovering from leg surgery. To be more precise, the woman's husband needed help, as he experienced difficulty cleaning and dressing his wife's wound. When Sister Carol arrived, she told him she needed water to disinfect his wife's leg, so she asked to see the faucet.

"Out this way, ma'am," the farmer said, leading her outside. To a barn. Sister Carol was confused.

"Where's the bucket?" she asked, guessing that's what they had come to retrieve.

"The bucket?" he asked. "The water. It's out here in the stable."

The husband explained that the house didn't have running water. He had been cleaning his wife's leg out in the barn. At a cow trough.

Sister Carol couldn't believe what she saw. She had been a resourceful and competent ER nurse. Yet here she was, looking at a man who used a cow trough to clean his wife's surgical wounds. Her skin crawled. But Carol put aside her judgment and transformed into nursing mode.

"Here," she said, pointing to a nearby pail. "Let's fill this bucket and bring it inside. We'll heat up the water. Then I'll show you how to clean and dress the wound."

Sister Carol arrived home later that night. She was covered in cobwebs, and the stench of farm animals lodged in her nostrils. Had she really given up a rewarding, albeit exhausting, career as an ER nurse for this? She scrubbed herself off and climbed into bed.

The next morning, Sister Carol asked her supervisor, "Where the hell did you send me last night?"

Smiling, her boss told her she would meet all kinds of people as a visiting nurse. Hospitals were one thing, but when people were home, they had to make use of available resources. Sister Carol's job was to help them figure it out—maybe not solve every problem, but at least throw them a lifeline. As for the case of the cow trough, the boss told Sister Carol that this experience in rural Illinois would help ease her into her next assignment. She would have to drive herself way out to Randolph County, where a young man lay dying, his parents tending to him in his childhood bedroom.

————

Before he became sick, when he was still toned and athletic, Carol's new patient had moved to New York City to pursue his dream of becoming a professional ballet dancer. He just couldn't see a future for himself in his small, conservative hometown. He didn't fit in, and like countless other men facing similar circumstances in the 1980s, he looked elsewhere to fulfill his dreams.

Carol's patient had struggled to find his footing when he arrived in New York, but he persevered and built a new life, step by step. His goal of becoming a professional dancer was realized when he landed a spot with the Joffrey Ballet. Everything seemed to be falling into place. But soon after, in a cruel twist of fate, he got sick. He managed for a while on his own, but when he became too weak to care for himself, he moved back home with his mom and dad. They were shocked when they laid eyes on him. His once muscular body was now frail. He looked aged and malnourished. Perhaps worst of all, his spirit seemed crushed.

Illness alone is bad enough. Terminal illness, even worse. And the patient's parents quickly learned three things, each adding a level of shock more traumatic than the next: Their son was gay. He had AIDS. And he had come home to die.

Back home, local hospitals had been reluctant to admit him. Doctors seemed scared of the unknown and in the early 1980s, little was understood about AIDS. Besides, they reasoned, what could medicine do? There was no cure, extended hospital stays were very expensive, nursing homes wanted nothing to do with the infected, and insurance companies fought claims.

The young man's parents, exhausted and unsure what they could do for their son, sought a nurse who could at least help alleviate some of his pain and discomfort. But this arrangement at first proved difficult. Even some battle-tested nurses feared being in the same room with him, never mind touching his open wounds or risking exposure to his contaminated blood. Those nurses offered the family their apologies, but no, they would not help. The parents remained steadfast in seeking care for their dying son. That's how they found Sister Carol.

She listened stoically as her boss briefed her about her new patient. She had been drawn to her religious order, the Hospital Sisters of Saint Francis, precisely because the sisters who ministered before her had toiled in hospitals in some of the most remote parts of the world. They opened and staffed clinics for the poor in rural Midwestern America, they sent missionary nurses to China in the 1920s, and they provided nursing care in Nagasaki following the US bombing in 1945. The sisters ministered in the spirit of their order's namesake, Saint Francis of Assisi, who cared for lepers in thirteenth-century Italy. Confronting the reality of working with a patient with AIDS, Sister Carol turned to Saint Francis for strength.

But this would not be Sister Carol's first brush with a dangerous disease. Back when she was a nursing student, she was assigned a patient requiring long-term care. A few weeks went by when one of the older nurses, who had read up on Carol's patient, approached her.

"Why aren't you wearing more protective clothing when you enter the room?" the nurse asked Sister Carol, who shrugged. The thought had not crossed her mind.

"You know he has tuberculosis, right?" the nurse said.

Carol hadn't known that about her patient, in fact, but she was unfazed, under the impression that this was just part of the job. Sisters go where they are needed, and this patient needed her.

Now, a couple of decades later, Sister Carol found herself face-to-face with another sick patient. She could not wrap her head around why others had refused him care.

"As a nurse, as a sister, why wouldn't I care for someone?" she asked. "I mean, they're sick, they're a person, they're a child of God. Why wouldn't I care for them?"

A willingness to help was one thing, but Carol's patient was suffering from a disease she simply did not understand. She was unsure what kind of care he needed. She asked around, but her colleagues provided few answers. Carol grew frustrated but decided to focus on comfort care. She brought her patient water, cleaned him, and administered basic pain medication.

Eager to help her patient's parents with the endless maze of health-care bureaucracy, Sister Carol transformed into something akin to a social worker. She accompanied them to appointments and harangued insurance company reps to process payments. She made sure the young man received needed drugs and medical devices. She sat with him as he slept, then changed his sweat-soaked sheets when he awoke. It was exhausting work, always an uphill climb, and she felt that people were almost going out of their way to make a young man's final days as difficult as possible. Perhaps trying to make up for the lack of medical options available, she promised she would learn everything she could about this new disease. Her pledge, however, came too late for this particular family. Carol's first patient with AIDS died just two weeks after she met him.

Carol took comfort in knowing that her patient's suffering had come to an end, but that comfort was short-lived as she confronted the immediate problem of how to handle his remains. She had read that hospitals, afraid of contamination, sometimes used black garbage bags to discard the bodies of patients who had died from AIDS-related complications. Some funeral homes refused to care for the remains, fearful both of infection and reputation. Carol again went beyond her official duties as a homecare nurse, helping her patient's parents properly bury their son.

———

In debriefing the case with her boss, Sister Carol said she hadn't been prepared to care for the patient. At this point, in 1984, about three hundred thousand Americans had been living with HIV, government public health officials later estimated, but medical professionals even in places with large gay populations such as New York and San Francisco were still challenged by the intricacies of this little-understood disease. What hope was there, she asked, for a small-town homecare nurse like herself?

"We need more education," Sister Carol explained. "Especially if we're going to start seeing more cases."

Over the next several months, Sister Carol tried on her own to learn more. The county health department held a workshop. Sister Carol went. The state health department offered training. Carol attended. She made calls to nurses and doctors over in St. Louis. They told her all they knew, but it simply wasn't enough.

One night during dinner, in 1986, Sister Carol told her friend and colleague Sister Mary Ellen Rombach about her encounters with people suffering from HIV and AIDS. She explained how frustrated she was that she couldn't do more to help the young men in their agonizing final weeks. There had only been a few patients, but their stories had burned themselves into Carol's memory.

As she listened, Sister Mary Ellen's eyes grew wide. She hadn't realized that Sister Carol's caseload had included patients with HIV and AIDS. In Sister Mary Ellen's role as a chaplain at their religious order's hospital, Saint Elizabeth's, she had encountered a couple of patients with HIV. Their families seemed beyond her capacity to comfort. These were unpleasant feelings for experienced nuns who felt like they had seen it all. As Sister Mary Ellen told Sister Carol about her experiences at the hospital, they were both shocked by the similarities in their work. They were determined to do more, but they needed help.

Sister Mary Ellen had an idea. She had a gay nephew in Atlanta who worked in medicine. Mary Ellen called him to see if he had any thoughts as to how she and Sister Carol could learn more about providing care and compassion to people with AIDS. He told his aunt that if she and Carol were serious, they needed to go somewhere they could see firsthand the medical and social horror of the disease. They should figure out a way to meet with the communities suffering the most. The pair of nuns knew this meant they had to get out of Belleville.

First, they headed to Kansas City, a four-hour journey during which they talked about recent cases and created a list of questions about AIDS care. Sister Carol was particularly interested in learning more about how HIV and AIDS affected mental health, thinking back to a patient she had encountered at Saint Elizabeth's, in his twenties, weak and suffering from hallucinations. A nurse had found him running through the hallways, naked, screaming about terrifying images only he could see. Not knowing what else to do, the staff admitted him to the psychiatric ward.

"Surely there's a better way," Carol had thought.

Once they arrived in Kansas City, the nuns visited the Good Samaritan House, a local organization that provided AIDS hospice care. The house consisted of six bedrooms where many people with AIDS spent their final days. The local Catholic Charities agency volunteered its tax-exempt status to the project so the house could engage in fundraising. Carol and Mary Ellen, eager to get to work back home in Belleville, thought a hospice house might be a welcome addition.

The staff members in Kansas City explained how they tried to meet the needs of their clients and how the hospice worked in partnership with the local community. Carol and Mary Ellen met some of the residents, sharing meals and listening to their struggles. They spent the night, the first time they slept in a place that people with AIDS called home. As they packed up and prepared for the ride back to Belleville the next morning, they apprehensively chatted about their lodging.

"Do you think somebody with AIDS slept in that bed?" Sister Carol asked Sister Mary Ellen. "Or *died*, right here?"

They couldn't wait to get home to shower. Carol told me she and Mary Ellen weren't necessarily scared of contracting HIV, but that the gravity of the situation weighed heavily on them. They knew the other nuns would be afraid when they returned to their shared house, especially when they explained the sleeping arrangements.

I have my doubts about some of the ways Sister Carol frames this history. In some ways, she is difficult to read. She's a natural storyteller, supplying plenty of details and quotes and always landing the story just so. But when I ask about how experiences like spending a night in an AIDS hospice challenged or changed her, she tends to clam up. She says she never had problems with gay people, that she didn't harbor biases or preconceived ideas about their lives.

"Did you know many gay men before you started your AIDS work?" I ask.

"No, not really," she tells me.

How then, I wonder, was she so certain that she held no biased opinions about gay people? The more we talk, however, the more I realize that the details of her transformation from a small-town nun to an advocate for gay men, IV drug users, and sex workers can be found just as much in the pauses as in the fact-filled stories themselves.

———

Sister Carol and Sister Mary Ellen had been impressed with the Good Samaritan House, but they still had many unanswered questions. They had each seen just a few patients with HIV and they felt it was only a matter of time before the number of cases grew back home in Belleville. They decided to seek out more answers up north in Chicago, home to one of the nation's largest gay populations. They needed a fixer of sorts, someone who could make appointments and show them the ropes. A nun from their order living in Chicago connected them with Father Bob Rybicki.

Father Rybicki was in his thirties, but he had already become a leader in HIV and AIDS care in the Chicago area. He led the clinical program at the Howard Brown Health Center, which served primarily lesbians and gays. Father Rybicki patiently answered Carol and Mary Ellen's many questions about how HIV and AIDS were affecting the gay community. But the young priest also had the foresight to recognize that the two nuns should be aware that all populations were vulnerable to HIV. So he brought Carol and Mary Ellen to a local hospital that specialized in treating women with HIV and AIDS, many of them sex workers. He hammered the point that stigma of any kind had no place in illness but acknowledged that fighting stigma was an uphill battle. Father Rybicki told the nuns to be aware of how widespread societal views, with their power to infect the outlook of even well-meaning people, could find their way into their own subconscious motivations.

"When it comes to adults with AIDS," he would say to anyone who listened, "the most common perception still is that you are dealing with a sinner. 'Was this person gay, promiscuous, a drug user?'"

That attitude, he believed, seemed to affect everyone's views on HIV and AIDS. If Carol and Mary Ellen were serious about working in this field, Father Rybicki told them, they had to look at their own prejudices and biases—and then strive to overcome them. It was a lesson Carol would hear again and again as she continued to seek out others who could help her learn.

By the end of her visit, Sister Carol was awed at the availability of resources in Chicago, both in terms of ministry and healthcare offerings, for people with HIV and AIDS. She and Sister Mary Ellen talked the whole way home. Whatever hesitations they may have harbored after Kansas City were gone. They knew they had found their calling, and they spent the next few weeks thinking of how they could acquire the skills and know-how they needed to minister and nurse more effectively.

"I didn't know where, I didn't know how, I didn't know when, but I knew this is what I was called to do," Sister Mary Ellen recalled later. "And I knew it with a certainty that I've never known anything else."

But as members of a religious community, they needed permission when it came to making future plans. Sister Carol and Sister Mary Ellen would have to convince their superiors that AIDS was an illness their order should take seriously and that they were the ones to lead the effort. After spending time in prayer, confident in their aspirations, they approached their religious superior—who looked at them like they were nuts.

"You want to do *what*?" she asked.

"We want to work with the gay community so we can learn how to care for people with AIDS," Sister Carol said, as if this were a routine request from two small-town nuns. "Oh, and we want to do it all in New York." Spending a few months in New York City, they reasoned, was the only way they could learn about the havoc caused by AIDS and connect with the people whose lives were routinely being turned upside down.

Their religious superior was skeptical, though not necessarily of their desire to help with HIV and AIDS. Sisters had always pitched in where there was a need, and New York was ground zero for this particular epidemic. It was just that Sister Carol always seemed ready to jump into a new project before completing her current mission. She had requested to become a homecare nurse and her superiors allowed it, so shouldn't she stick with that for a bit? Sister Carol also tended to push boundaries, and given the tension that existed in the church around the issue of homosexuality, the possibilities for conflict seemed endless. Plus, she had never even visited New York, much less lived there. It all seemed like too much.

"Let me think about it," their superior told them. "But in the meantime, put together a plan and lay out how you'll learn the skills you're seeking. Then come back to me."

Thrilled that their idea wasn't immediately rejected, Sister Carol and Sister Mary Ellen got to work. They remembered that a former executive at Saint Elizabeth's, their hospital in Belleville, had relocated to New York to manage a struggling Catholic hospital. Partly because of that hospital's mission, which included caring for those with no other place to go, and partly because of the influx of government money that would come in caring for people with AIDS, Saint Clare's Hospital in Hell's Kitchen became one of the first centers in New York to offer comprehensive AIDS care. Sister Mary Ellen called their former colleague and asked if she and Carol might come to New York for some sort of immersive internship.

"Absolutely," he said, eager to have two highly trained nuns with medical backgrounds assist his staff. "Give me a week and we'll figure it out."

The nuns met again with their supervisor and presented their plans. They would leave Belleville and spend about six months in New York, living in a Hell's Kitchen convent near the hospital with a group of other sisters. As for their work, they would split their time between Saint Clare's and Saint Vincent's Hospital, another Catholic institution, located in Greenwich Village, just a few miles south. Both hospitals cared for large patient populations of gay men with AIDS. When they weren't working in the hospitals, Sister Carol and Sister Mary Ellen planned to learn as much as possible about the gay community by attending workshops and volunteering on an AIDS hotline. Nothing would be off limits for the sisters, whose mission was to learn as much as possible in New York in order to help patients back in Belleville, where the full fury of AIDS was still off on the horizon.

The supervisor took a deep breath. She seemed to be taking her time before giving her answer. Sister Carol and Sister Mary Ellen braced for the worst.

"Sure, go for it," she said finally.

The pair of nuns got packing.

———

A few years after my first interview with Carol, I read through my transcript of our conversation. I wanted to make sure I caught every detail she shared with me. The recording amused me—listening to Carol speed through her stories, the clacking of my keyboard as I raced to keep up. Eventually I would convince Carol to slow down a bit, and I trusted that the audio recorder would catch everything. But something on the final page of the transcript suddenly caught my eye. Right before we hung up, Carol mentioned that a name had just popped into her head.

"Check out a Father William Hart McNichols," she told me. "He was an artist, and I remember being moved by his work on AIDS."

According to the transcript, I thanked Carol for the names and stories. I promised that I would be in touch and I added the artist's name to the growing list of people I needed to contact, but I didn't think much of it. I would come to learn that each story I researched led to another handful of stories, with people I interviewed supplying a few more names I should contact.

I wished I could have called everyone on that list, but at some point, at the urging of one of my colleagues, I had to stop reporting and focus on the stories at hand. Though Carol's suggestion sounded somewhat interesting—a priest and an artist working in HIV and AIDS care—I wanted to talk to people who were in the trenches. Not a quiet artist, squirreled away in a studio while others did the difficult work of healing and ministering and burying.

Eventually I'd learn, however, as had so many other headstrong young Catholics before me, that I should heed the advice of savvy Catholic sisters.

4

"IT HAS TO BE
A GAY PERSON"

Father Bill had just been ordained on a May day in 1979 when his dad invited him downstairs for a celebratory drink.

"Willy," his dad said, "I want to tell you a story."

Father Bill had grown up in a prominent Colorado political family. His grandfather was Denver's auditor, his uncle was the mayor, and his dad was lieutenant governor before he became governor in 1956. Bill remembers living in the governor's mansion as a young child. He met President John F. Kennedy.

Bill knew the family stories well, but not the one his dad would tell him that evening. As a young child, Bill's dad had witnessed members of Colorado's powerful Ku Klux Klan erect a cross on his lawn and set it on fire. His grandmother took Bill's dad out onto the porch, pointed to the masks the men wore, and said in a voice loud enough for them to hear, "They're all cowards. Don't ever be afraid of people who aren't willing to show who they are."

The story Bill listened to that night was another lesson from a family that had long taught him the importance of standing on the side of justice—a piece of advice that Bill had already practiced for years.

As a seminarian in Missouri in the 1970s, Bill was inspired by Catholics who had taken a firm stance against the Vietnam War. He joined a group of twenty-six other young Jesuits intent on ridding themselves of their draft exemption status as a way to protest. Their anti-war stance landed them in the pages of the *St. Louis Post-Dispatch*. He was just a kid, with thick, square-framed glasses and shaggy hair.

When Father Bill returned to Denver after ordination, he was artist-in-residence at the Jesuit-run Regis University. While there, a group called Dignity approached him. Founded in California in 1969 by Father Patrick Nidorf, Dignity consisted primarily of gay and lesbian Catholics who met for Mass and social activities in Catholic parishes. By the 1980s, the organization had expanded to local chapters throughout the country. Though Dignity was independent of the institutional church, its leaders maintained relationships with bishops and invited priests to celebrate Mass. Bill was impressed by Dignity's devotion to the church, and he recognized its precarious situation. Gay and lesbian Catholics were welcome to attend Mass, but the church taught that homosexuality was a sin. Wishing to show solidarity, he accepted their invitation.

Though a priest, Father Bill also wanted to become a professional artist, which meant pursuing more education. Not content to stay in Denver, and after gaining the approval of his Jesuit superiors, he applied to art school. When the Pratt Institute accepted him, he was elated. Like many young people intent on fulfilling their creative dreams, he headed to New York.

Father Bill's decision to pursue advanced studies in art was motivated in part by his desire to evangelize. This was a time when religious education was changing. Gone were the old days of the Baltimore Catechism, with straightforward, black-and-white lessons beginning with, "Question: Who made the world? Answer: God made the world." Suddenly, Catholics realized that children could be taught about their faith in the same ways they learned about other things, including the use of books specifically designed for kids. Bill had some early luck in this area, lending his illustrations to dozens of books about saints, Jesus and Mary, and churches. He felt he had found his footing after what had been a fairly difficult start in religious life.

Though his studies were meant to demand the bulk of his attention, Father Bill wasn't ready to give up face-to-face ministry. He loved being around people, listening to their hopes and struggles, and accompanying them as they sorted through life.

The needs he encountered were pressing. By 1983, a few years after Bill arrived in New York, more than three thousand Americans had been diagnosed with AIDS. The city's gay community was particularly hard hit. Leaders of Dignity's New York chapter recognized that its members had few outlets to process the growing epidemic, especially through a spiritual lens. They decided to host a Mass specifically for people with AIDS and their loved ones, and they approached Father Bill to ask if he would be willing to help. He loved working with Dignity, and the Masses would give him the opportunity to connect with other Catholics while earning money to pay his way in the Jesuit community. Yet he was torn over the invitation.

His focus was supposed to be his art. Every time he said yes to another commitment, that meant he devoted a bit less time to honing his craft. So as he had done since childhood, Bill turned to the lives of the saints for advice. He had recently read a book about Saint Damien of Molokai, a Belgian priest who ministered to Hawaiians suffering from leprosy in the late nineteenth century. Father Bill was shaken by Damien's story, amazed at his courage, and inspired by his commitment to the marginalized. Deeply spiritual, some might say mystical, Father Bill felt a pull from Father Damien.

"When I hung up the phone," he recalled of his conversation with Dignity, "I had a strong sense of Damien's presence, saying, 'You can't be afraid of this. This is why I've come into your life—to show you that the place of the Church is with people who are hurting, people who are sick, people whom other people are afraid of.'"

On the other hand, Father Bill knew that once he was involved in HIV and AIDS care, people would make assumptions about him, which brought up some painful memories from the time when he had first decided to be honest with others about his own inner life. Those painful memories lingered, and he worried that saying yes to the Mass might bring them to the surface. But he felt he had no choice. From the time he was a young child back in Denver, he had been taught to respond to suffering with compassion and to be courageous in the face of bullying.

———

At the AIDS Mass, Father Bill reminded the congregation that illness can never be interpreted as some sort of divine punishment. That was not just his personal opinion, he told those gathered; it was official church teaching.

Pointing to a church document outlining the sacrament of anointing the sick, sometimes called last rites, Bill said of illness, "while it is closely related to man's sinful condition, it cannot be understood as punishment which man suffers for his personal sins."

During the homily, the Rev. Mills Omaly, an Episcopal priest, talked about his own struggles with HIV and AIDS, lambasting the stigma that isolated people and perpetuated fear. (In less than a year, the forty-four-year-old Omaly would die from AIDS-related complications. Bill prayed for him at a later Mass.)

At the end of Mass, the nearly five hundred people in attendance were slow to leave. Hearing a Catholic priest acknowledge the reality of AIDS was powerful. Father Bill stayed to greet the worshippers, many of whom asked him questions: *Will you come visit my sick partner? My brother is ill and wants to be anointed. My cousin. My friend. My lover.*

Scattered throughout New York, the number of people with HIV and AIDS in need of spiritual care was growing. He said yes to as many requests as he thought feasible. He visited patients in the hospital during the day, hopping on the train to see others in their homes in Brooklyn, Queens, or sometimes even out in New Jersey. Late at night, when he finally returned home, he collapsed into bed, exhausted. As he thought about the young men, terrified of their illness and shunned by the world, he decided he had to reach more people. Here was a chance to minister to a community truly in need, one that seemed unable to catch a break. A community that Father Bill knew he must serve, because it was, after all, his own.

———

The first person with AIDS Father Bill ever visited on his own threw his world into chaos. He knew the patient was young, but the man's illness made him look decades older. On one side of the patient stood the man's mother and on the other side, his partner. Father Bill's mind flashed to the religious iconography that comprised so much of his spirituality. For a split second, he saw Christ, condemned by the world and dying on a cross, his anguished mother on one side and his beloved disciple on the other. It was so similar to what he saw in front of him. Father Bill was brought back to reality when he saw the patient's boyfriend dipping a straw into a small carton of orange juice. He held his finger over the top of the straw, trapping some of the juice, before releasing it into his partner's mouth.

"My God, he looks like a helpless baby bird," Bill thought to himself.

The image paralyzed Bill. All the seminary training, the hospice work, none of it had prepared him for this. His skills as a priest seemed useless in the face of so much suffering. He stammered, unsure what to say. As he left, he wondered: had he failed? Perhaps AIDS care was too much for this young Jesuit. Did the men afflicted with this awful disease, many of whom had faced discrimination from religious figures, even want help from a Catholic priest? How would he possibly conjure words of solace?

Father Bill wasn't sure, but he knew he had a duty to try. And he realized he had much more to learn.

He turned to the Gay Men's Health Crisis for answers to his questions. A small group of gay men had formed the organization in 1982 to empower the gay community to stand up for itself since so few others seemed interested in fighting AIDS. The first workshop Father Bill attended included about ten other people. Most were young like him, in their twenties and thirties, women and men who all wanted to help people with HIV and AIDS. The speakers that afternoon focused on education, as hysteria and misinformation about AIDS, and how it spread, were worsening the stigma facing people with the disease.

"What do you do if you're in the apartment of someone who has AIDS and they offer you a glass of water?" the presenter asked the group. "Is that safe?"

When nobody answered, the presenter told them it was fine. AIDS could not be spread by sharing utensils or dishes.

"What if you need to use the bathroom? Should you avoid touching doorknobs? How about sharing soap? Drying your hands with their towels, is that safe?"

The group nodded. The goal of the training was as simple as that, to inform people how HIV spread so those who wanted to help wouldn't worry about contracting the virus themselves. There were precautions volunteers should take, such as being careful with needles or open wounds. But in most situations, they would be safe. Fear served no purpose, especially when scientists were learning more about the virus with each passing week.

After the training, Father Bill formalized his ministry by volunteering regularly at Saint Vincent's Hospital in Greenwich Village. Located in the middle of a large population of gay New Yorkers, the Catholic hospital treated many patients with HIV and AIDS. Father Bill befriended the director of the hospital's pastoral care program, Sister Patrice Murphy, who was a fierce advocate for people with AIDS and a hero to many in the gay community. She met with Father Bill daily, outlining his responsibilities and helping him grow as a caregiver to people with AIDS. His tasks included visiting patients on the AIDS ward, a place that would become an epicenter of one of the deadliest pandemics in modern history.

————

As I learned more of Father Bill's story, I asked questions about some of the young men he had accompanied through their final days. Nearly all of them were gay, he told me, and most were Catholic. I could relate— at least to their backgrounds if not their suffering. I asked about their lives because I was curious whether Father Bill encountered resistance from any of the men he met when he first identified himself as a Catholic priest. After all, the dynamic between the institutional church and the gay community was fraught in the 1980s. In many ways, not much has changed. Surely some people were too angry to want Bill's help.

I'm privileged to know many gay priests. Some are open about their sexuality, letting the chips fall where they may, refusing to compromise for the sake of the institution. Others are more cautious, barely alluding to their sexuality but giving enough clues so that we can develop honest and healthy friendships. I try not to judge either way. The pressures gay

⸝s face from church leaders to keep their sexual orientation a secret, ⸝hile toeing the church's line on homosexuality, is enormous.

Still, I've had some negative encounters with priests when it comes to homosexuality, so I understand why many LGBT people don't feel welcome in the Catholic Church. I've met priests who seem fixated on the church's stance against homosexuality, letting it overtake their pastoral instincts. Then there's social media, which has a tendency to amplify the most strident voices, including clerics who believe homosexuality is part of Satan's plan to destroy humanity. Trolls have sent me more than my fair share of links to those kinds of messages. But for the most part, I've been extremely fortunate. My husband and I invited several priests to our wedding. My story is not one of being harmed by the church.

But many LGBT Catholics have experienced a different reality. I cannot really imagine what it must have been like for them in the 1980s, when their world was falling apart and their church regularly fought against their rights. On some occasions, church leaders suggested that gay men with HIV actually deserved to be sick. How did Father Bill manage to be a Catholic priest ministering to a community that felt under attack by the church? His answer turned out to be complicated.

Father Bill knew how others saw him, especially gay men and their partners who might already have been wary of receiving care in a Catholic hospital, surrounded by plentiful signs and symbols of what could be an antagonistic faith. To many men dying from AIDS, Bill represented an institution that judged and condemned them and considered their lives disordered. Bill was savvy enough to understand that if he were to provide any hope or solace to these men, he needed to establish a level of trust.

"I knew that people were so hostile about the church," he told me.

But he didn't blame them. He could see the hypocrisy as well as anyone. As a precaution, when visiting patients, he swapped out his black shirt and Roman collar for civilian clothes: a white shirt and a brown sport coat. The only clue that he was affiliated with the church was a small lapel pin, depicting Saint Anthony and the baby Jesus; he thought the image conveyed love. But you would have to stand pretty close to Bill to see the pin, and even then, the message might not be clear.

"Who are you?" a patient might ask.

"A chaplain."

"What kind of chaplain?"

"Catholic," Bill would say, his voice soft.

"You're a priest?"

"Yep, I am. I'm Bill."

By this point in the introduction, many patients relaxed. They could sense they had an ally in Father Bill. But not always.

Some might say, "Oh. I don't want a priest. Get the hell out of here."

And Bill would leave, adding, "I'm sorry. I'll be around if you need anything."

In those moments, Father Bill felt rejected. But he understood the anger because even though he held a special place in his heart for people with AIDS, he recognized the wider church was hostile to gays and lesbians. If only the church would listen to gay men and their loved ones, Bill lamented.

"I've encountered so many AIDS patients who have found light in their illness, and made others see it," he thought. "The church will come around when it discovers that there are gay people who have lived full Christian lives and faced death with courage."

———

Father Bill's desire to help people with HIV and AIDS was motivated by more than a general orientation toward caring for the sick. I knew that he was openly gay before he and I connected the first time. And once we started talking, we were pretty candid with one another about our lives.

From my vantage point, Father Bill seemed well adjusted and comfortable identifying as a gay priest. This made sense given his embrace of Dignity and his early entry into AIDS ministry. As I mentioned, I've seen how some priests struggle around how much to reveal about their sexuality to other people. Bill just wasn't like that. When it came to talking to people with AIDS, he thought being honest about his own sexual orientation was the best way to forge an authentic connection. Gay priests, he decided, had a unique role to play in the AIDS crisis.

"I felt healing was needed," he said. "It has to be a gay person. We have to bring healing to each other."

But simply having that insight didn't make the reality of living as a gay priest much easier.

By the end of the 1980s, Bill had told several of his friends and colleagues that he was gay. But when New Ways Ministry, a group that ministered to gay and lesbian Catholics in the church, asked Bill to write about his experience for a book chronicling gay priests, he hedged. Coming out publicly in a book would invite abuse, like when he opened his mailbox and found pieces of hate mail. More importantly to Father Bill, coming out publicly could negatively affect his AIDS ministry if his superiors became uncomfortable with his increasingly public profile. The reality was simple: gay people did not have a home in the Catholic Church. Even the head of the Catholic bishops' conference in 1987, who was considered a moderate on the subject, suggested gay Catholics try to "switch" and become straight.

Even with all the uncertainty weighing on him, Father Bill decided the benefits of coming out were greater than the risks. He wanted to do everything he could to let the many gay people he met through his ministry know they had a place in the church and an ally in Bill.

New Ways Ministry's leaders knew they were putting Father Bill in an uncomfortable situation. There were a handful of other openly gay Catholic priests in the United States at the time, but coming out publicly had put their careers at risk. The organization offered Father Bill the opportunity to publish under a pseudonym. He would have none of it. He understood the kindness behind the gesture, but to him, anonymity implied shame, and homosexuality was not something he thought had to lurk in the shadows.

"If I'm going to write, it has to be under my own name," Bill told them. "Otherwise, what effect will it have? What's the point of coming out in the church if I'm not going to put my own name on it?"

Accepting the invitation to write the chapter, however, wasn't something Bill could do unilaterally. As a young Jesuit priest, he needed permission from his superiors, which meant initiating what he suspected would be an uncomfortable conversation. Bill called his superior, the provincial of the Missouri province of the Society of Jesus. He explained why he thought it was important for him to come out publicly. His superior listened carefully and asked thoughtful follow-up questions. After Bill laid out his case, the provincial told Bill that the decision was his to make. The Jesuits wouldn't stand in his way.

"But if you come out, you will be unavailable to work at a Jesuit high school, college, or parish."

Though subtle, and delivered with kindness, the implication was ugly. Father Bill was being told he could come out, but as a gay man, he wouldn't be allowed to minister to children or even young adults. Bill, determined not to let other people's fear drag him down, said he wasn't offended by the response. In fact, it gave him the freedom to do what he wanted. He was an illustrator. He worked at the hospital. Neither of those jobs would be in jeopardy if he wrote the chapter. Plus, he thought that most people already assumed he was gay anyway. Any man who worked in the AIDS arena at the time seemed to be gay, he felt. He decided to write the chapter.

"Homosexuality in the Priesthood and the Religious Life" was published in 1989. Bill's chapter isn't terribly long, just eight pages. He lays out his argument clearly: gay people have a place in the church, including the priesthood. But what is most remarkable about Bill's essay is that he did not present his sexuality as a cross to bear or as something to overcome so that he could live an authentically Christian life, an emerging ethos in the church at that time. Catholic teaching did not go as far as some more conservative Christian denominations in saying that a homosexual orientation itself was a sin. Instead, Catholic moral teaching condemned sexual acts between two people of the same sex. "We are all sinners," some Catholics would say in an effort to appear more welcoming to gay and lesbian people. In this view, each of us deserved mercy and forgiveness; homosexuality was just one sin among many others.

But Father Bill rejected this theology. He wrote that his sexuality was a gift from God and even "a component of the priesthood formed for me by Jesus." He didn't have much trouble reconciling being a priest and being gay. "For me personally, it would be no more difficult to balance or to integrate being gay and priest than being a priest and artist, or priest and teacher, or priest and retreat director," he wrote.

At the same time, Father Bill didn't shy away from naming the source of some challenges he faced as a gay Catholic priest: the church itself. He combined his own experiences with the insights of the gay and lesbian people to whom he ministered through Dignity, the partners of the gay men dying in hospitals, and even the activists who took on the church. Most of the difficulty, he asserted, came from "the relentless violence and persecution of religions and societies."

Father Bill felt he had a duty to speak up and use his platform to stand in solidarity with gay men who suffered from callous indifference or outright abuse when they revealed they were sick with AIDS. He felt especially impassioned to denounce those who sought to portray AIDS as an outburst of divine wrath, a belief espoused by some Catholic leaders. "Dark days have descended as the accusers now point to a disease that is supposed to have been sent by God to infect gay people," he wrote. "The accusation is that God finds gay men so repulsive that God seeks to eliminate them."

In the 1980s, it was rare for a priest to say something affirming about homosexuality, much less describe it as a gift from God that helped his priesthood. But Father Bill didn't stop there. He sought to redirect any positive attention he might receive about his own bravery in coming out as gay toward the plight of people with HIV and AIDS. He acknowledged walking alongside them was not easy work. "I do not pretend for a moment that I have been able to walk stoically in and out of the world of this disease," he wrote. "For the first six months, at least, I left hospitals and apartments in a kind of numbing fog."

Many people working in HIV and AIDS care, including doctors and nurses, priests and nuns, were being "confronted, often for the first time, with gay people as human beings," Father Bill witnessed through his hospital ministry. These interactions, the accompaniment from life to illness to death, led to a greater awareness about the humanity of gay people and those they loved. "The coldhearted prejudice, either intellectual or visceral, is being shattered by the truth people witness," he added.

But what an unjust price to force the gay community to pay for greater understanding from society.

5

CATHOLIC TO THE BONES

A sticky note on a newspaper article changed the life of David Pais. Even though I work in journalism, it was difficult for me to appreciate the impact of a relatively short story on an entire generation of gay men. I had previously read this article, but it wasn't until I met David that I began to appreciate how those 898 words heralded the beginnings of something that unleashed a terrifying new era.

David had moved to New York as a young man and created a vibrant life for himself. Though New York had its challenges, it was hard to think of a place more accepting for gays and lesbians. The bars and bookstores provided a sense that it wasn't only normal to be gay but exciting and even cutting edge. It was the Fourth of July, 1981, and a friend had slid a clipping from the previous day's *New York Times* under the door of David's Greenwich Village apartment. Those feelings of limitless possibility were halted, for a brief moment anyway, with that article.

David and his neighbor, Donald, had a mutual acquaintence, a man named Paul, who had become sick, seemingly out of nowhere, before he suddenly died. The circumstances of the illness had remained something of a mystery. Paul had been young and healthy when his strength seemed to vanish almost overnight. But that morning in July, the note from Donald finally offered some insight.

"This is what Paul died from."

Curious, David peeled back the note and began reading the article.

"Rare cancer seen in 41 homosexuals," blared the headline in all capital letters. The *Times* wasn't known for its robust coverage of gay issues, so that the story made it into the paper at all was remarkable. David kept reading.

"Doctors in New York and California have diagnosed among homosexual men 41 cases of a rare and often rapidly fatal form of cancer," he read. "Eight of the victims died less than 24 months after the diagnosis was made."

The article explained what doctors knew about the disease, which at this point wasn't much. The cancer was Kaposi's sarcoma (KS), which often presented itself in the form of small, dark spots appearing on the legs. A person could normally live with the disease for about a decade before it became fatal. But the article explained that in these few dozen cases, the purple lesions attacked the bodies of previously healthy young men, sometimes at first being mistaken for bruises or blemishes. Lymph nodes became inflamed, and patients died in a matter of months, far faster than the typical course. The article implied that the afflicted men used drugs during sex and that many of them had a history of contracting sexually transmitted diseases. Doctors speculated that the cancer was not contagious, and the article said it posed little threat "outside the homosexual community." But a cancer affecting only gay men? It just didn't make sense.

Just a few weeks later, David's neighbor was also diagnosed with KS. Donald was creative, bright, articulate, handsome, and kind. The total package. Like other young, liberated gay men who seemed to have it all, he could also be a bit self-absorbed. Who wasn't in the 1980s New York gay scene? But when Donald was diagnosed with this cancer, David saw him change dramatically. He lost weight and splotches appeared. But more striking were the emotional and even spiritual transformations.

"Between July and November, I saw this vibrant young man morph into the closest example of sainthood I had ever seen," David told me.

Knowing the fear that accompanied an illness with so much uncertainty, Donald told his doctors that they should refer any other young men with similar diagnoses to him. He would gladly answer their questions about his own experience with the illness, pass along information and helpful tips, and even just listen to their worries. It was a kind of ministry, even if Donald didn't view it quite that way. But to David, who was Catholic to the bones, this was a moment of transformative grace in action. He watched his neighbor throw off the vanity of his youth and become a source of compassion for others.

Donald died in November 1981. David vowed then and there that he would do whatever he could to help gay men battling this deadly cancer.

———

Learning Sister Carol's and Father Bill's stories helped me understand the history of how the Catholic Church, or at least parts of it, interacted with the LGBT community in a wholly new way. But their insights could take me only so far. Though they are both approachable and generous with their time, I can relate to a priest and a nun only up to a certain point before the distance between our life experiences becomes too great. I was curious for another perspective. I wanted to know what life was like for gay Catholics living in a big city in the 1980s, how they navigated dating and going to church. What were they thinking when church leaders attacked gay civil rights bills? Why did they stay Catholic at all? Such questions eventually led me to David.

A gentle man in his seventies who has endured more trauma than his kind demeanor lets on, David is slightly balding and sports a thick gray beard and mustache. He keeps a stuffed Snoopy on his desk at work. We met at his office at the Gay Men's Health Crisis (GMHC), the organization that decades earlier had helped Father Bill learn about HIV and AIDS. I would not learn until much later how David's and Bill's stories overlapped, one of many surprising coincidences I would discover during this project.

I already knew a bit about GMHC, mostly through what I had read about the early AIDS activist Larry Kramer and how he portrayed the organization in his play *The Normal Heart*, which I had seen a few years earlier. David filled me in on the rest of the story as we walked through the office. He seemed to know everyone on the predominantly young staff, stopping by desks to say hello and introducing me as a Catholic journalist working on a project about AIDS. When we arrived back at his office, I asked permission to record our conversation. He said, "Absolutely."

———

Just a couple of months following the death of his neighbor, David learned that the newly formed Gay Men's Health Crisis was distributing information about the mysterious new plague that had been described so vaguely in the *Times*. The organization's first "office" was an answering machine set up in the living room of an early volunteer. More than a hundred people called that first night, showing how desperately the gay community needed information about this disease. When David learned that GMHC needed help, he volunteered immediately, one of several gay Catholics to help the organization early on, assistance that included a sizable donation from Dignity's New York chapter.

Answering questions about the dangers of AIDS and encouraging people to protect themselves seemed right up David's alley. So he headed to the group's new headquarters, located in the basement of a brownstone on Twenty-Second Street, where a folding table, metal chair, and telephone awaited him. The calls from terrified gay men, scared and seeking any helpful information, seemed endless. Was this a new sexually transmitted disease? Could I get it through kissing or sharing drinks? How will I know if I have it?

It became clear, however, that answering individual questions on a telephone was not the most efficient way to spread information about AIDS. Organizers decided a town hall-style meeting made sense. But where? The brownstone basement certainly wasn't big enough and there wasn't enough money to rent a large venue. David had an idea. He regularly attended Mass at Saint Joseph's in the Village, with ample space, including a parochial school nearby. David told the priests about his volunteering and mentioned the predicament about finding space. He asked if the parish had a room they could spare.

"Of course," they said, offering the school gym.

The day of the meeting arrived. Seats quickly filled up and people were still walking in. The gym proved to be too small and, not wanting to turn anyone away, the organizers asked if they could move the meeting into the church. The request was bold, but so was GMHC. They wanted to host a forum about how to make gay sex safer in the era of this new disease—inside a building affiliated with an institution that regularly fought against the rights of gay people. One that taught that gay sex was not only unsafe but a sin. Would there be conflict? What if parishioners found out? Would the men attending the meeting even be willing to go inside?

But the priests at Saint Joe's put all those worries aside and lent the church to GMHC. About six hundred people filed into the sanctuary, ready for a raucous conversation about how to slow the spread of the disease.

"People weren't used to hearing very honest and direct statements coming from community educators," David recalled. And even when surrounded by stained glass windows and a towering image of Christ, the group did not mince words. Attendees shouted questions about how to make sex safer, whether condoms were effective, if some sex acts were less risky than others. The speakers recognized the need to disseminate accurate information and answered the questions with clarity.

"The first public education program about AIDS that was ever held in Greenwich Village was held inside a Catholic church," David told me in his office, beaming, proud of the parish for stepping up and serving a community in need.

David was encouraged that his church had done the right thing in this instance—but he was uncertain about this relationship's durability.

In the months after the town hall at Saint Joseph's, David continued to volunteer at GMHC. He saw the power of putting information in the hands of people who were otherwise underinformed and afraid. Recalling how his neighbor had shown such grit in helping to educate other people, David was motivated to do what he could to help. He was inspired when one day he saw a lively Catholic nun come by GMHC for training about HIV and AIDS. He learned later that Sister Patrice Murphy was the head of pastoral care at Saint Vincent's. It made him feel good to see other Catholics stepping up to help people with AIDS, especially when there was so much negativity from some church leaders about homosexuality—and near silence about the growing epidemic.

For David, the stream of endless suffering became inescapable. The calls he answered often came from anxious and scared men. The people he visited in hospitals were so similar to him, having moved to New York to chase their dreams. But they now lay dying, often in pain and suffering from emotional trauma. Too many of his friends had been diagnosed with AIDS, and David felt helpless as each one became weak. So many of them eventually died, cutting short any opportunities to grapple with grief. It was all becoming too much. He needed to step away from volunteering and focus on caring for himself.

David was dating a man named Bill who lived in Philadelphia, and it was around this time that they decided to move in together. Originally from Long Island, Bill was an accountant and ready to get back to New York. David and Bill were in love and building their lives together when groups like GMHC suggested that gay men be tested regularly for HIV. People who tested positive had few options in terms of treatment at that point; the virus would run its course and they could develop AIDS. But a test would at least give them vital information so they could take steps to slow the spread of the virus. Men who knew they were HIV-positive could insist on condoms when having sex and let previous partners know of their status.

David and Bill decided it was responsible to be tested, and given David's involvement with HIV and AIDS education, they wanted to lead by example. So they were tested and readied themselves for any bad news that might follow. Then a wallop: David and Bill each tested positive for HIV. David's T-cell count was higher than 200 and he was not experiencing opportunistic infections, so while he was HIV-positive, he did not have AIDS. Bill's T-cell count was just 60. David's partner was extremely sick.

In the days and weeks following their diagnoses, emotions swirled in David's head. He wasn't sure what to do, how to act, what to say. But he knew faith had to play a role in their response. Bill had been raised Methodist, but he wasn't particularly active in any church. After his diagnosis, he wanted to find an affirming faith community. David liked Saint Joe's, but he had decided his life would now be devoted to caring for Bill. He sought to be a supportive, loving partner. So together they found a place where they both felt welcome, Saint John's Episcopal Church, and David saw Bill thrive.

For the next two years, David prayed he could become the partner Bill needed by providing love, support, and compassion during a particularly trying time. He joined a group at GMHC for men whose partners were dying from AIDS. He learned what to expect and met people in similar situations. But David's journey was just beginning.

6

"AN INTRINSIC MORAL EVIL"

Around one thousand people gathered inside Saint Francis Xavier Church for more than an hour on a Saturday night in March 1987. Located just a short walk from both Greenwich Village and Chelsea, the parish was home to a large cohort of gay and lesbian Catholics and the site of a weekly Mass hosted by Dignity. Normally these gatherings were joyful occasions. But tonight, melancholy permeated the celebration. Father Bill McNichols, exhausted from visiting ever-increasing numbers of people with AIDS, nonetheless made his way to the church, one of several priests on hand to mark a sad and historic moment.

Throughout the nation, bishops evicted Dignity chapters from Catholic spaces, part of the church's crackdown on gay and lesbian activism. Shortly before Christmas in 1986, the chapter in Syracuse was told they could no longer gather at a Catholic church. Then the same story played out in Atlanta, Cincinnati, Minneapolis. And now, New York. Word had come from the chancery about ten days earlier: Over the objections of the

Jesuits who ran the parish, Dignity would no longer be allowed to celebrate Mass at Saint Francis Xavier. Cardinal O'Connor told the media of his decision: "There are divine laws which give us life," and as Catholics, "we don't believe that they can be changed." Tonight, however, gay and lesbian Catholics in New York would refuse to go quietly into the night. This was a Mass of defiance.

Emotions ran high. After communion, one worshipper stopped in front of a statue of the Virgin Mary. Looking up at her, he fell to his knees and began to cry.

The congregation listened to a speech from the president of Dignity's New York chapter. "Tonight we are not leaving a church behind," he said. "Instead we are taking a church with us. Tonight, our right to be in this building does not end, because no one, not even a pope or a pompous cardinal, can take away our baptismal right." He added that gay Catholics were everywhere in the church, not part of some fringe. "We are your priests, your nuns, your religious brothers. We run and staff your schools, colleges, and hospitals. We are your social workers, your accountants, and your janitors. And, no doubt, we even make your fancy robes, Cardinal O'Connor," he said. "But in spite of all this, we stand here tonight and say loudly and clearly, we are not going away." Worshippers stood on their kneelers and cheered.

With candles in hand, evoking the AIDS vigils now held in cities throughout the world, the crowd walked down the long center aisle at the end of Mass. As they turned their backs to the altar to process toward the exit, some looked up at the dome high above the congregation. Others glanced around at the side chapels, one with a statue of Saint Aloysius Gonzaga, the sixteenth-century Jesuit who died while ministering during an earlier plague. This was the last time many of them would be inside a building that had become their spiritual home. They sang "We Shall Overcome." As they processed out, the church darkened, the candlelight now outside, illuminating the heart of a community suffering from HIV and AIDS. The large congregation yelled into the night, "We are the church!"

They walked four blocks to the Lesbian and Gay Community Services Center. This space lacked the grandeur of Saint Francis Xavier, but the members of Dignity felt welcome there.

Father Bill joined the march. Besieged by emotions, he wondered how he could help this community now, given the church's hostility to gay people at such a delicate moment. In an interview airing on ABC News, he said plainly why gay Catholics were so angry at church leaders.

"I think it is the cruelest thing in the world to ask a human being never to be touched, never to be held, never to be treated like everyone else gets treated, simply because they're born one way or another. They ask that of no other person."

Though his voice in the video is meek, the words are bold, a young priest very publicly standing up to a powerful institution.

––––––––

The vigil that night was a culmination of years of tension between the Church and the gay community. By 1986, more than twenty-four thousand Americans had died from AIDS. Though Catholics were by this point already engaged in HIV and AIDS ministry in several US cities, the institutional church was still largely silent when it came to the epidemic. Even five years into the disease, Pope John Paul II had not publicly addressed HIV or AIDS. Individual US bishops had commented on the crisis, but their national association had not released any major documents, which could have mobilized the church's vast healthcare and education systems. What was now a global crisis simply wasn't capturing the attention of the church in any systemic manner. That all began to change in October 1986—though not in the way that many gay Catholics had hoped.

Newspapers throughout the United States reported on Halloween Day that the Vatican had promulgated a letter to bishops around the world earlier that month on the question of homosexuality. Cardinal Joseph Ratzinger, who two decades later would become Pope Benedict XVI, was head of the Congregation for the Doctrine of the Faith. He had drafted the letter to rearticulate the church's ban on gay sex, but also to condemn a homosexual orientation itself, along with what he called "deceitful propaganda" that urged the church to accept its gay members with love. The "Halloween letter," as it became known in gay circles, was about more than theology. Pointedly, it was written in English, making clear that its intended audience was US Catholics. Its unnamed target, in fact, was Dignity. This letter launched a series of events leading to Dignity's expulsion from Saint Francis Xavier and other Catholic churches throughout the United States.

The letter was in some ways a response to an earlier Vatican teaching, released in 1975, that concerned sexual ethics. The views expressed then seemed somewhat progressive compared to fundamentalist Christian churches, because the Vatican differentiated between homosexual actions, which it called sinful, and homosexual orientation, which remained a mystery and thus morally neutral. "Love the sinner, hate the sin," in other words. (This language would one day bother Catholics on the front lines of the AIDS crisis, but for the time, it seemed better than simply, "hate the sinner.") The 1975 document led some popular Catholic theologians and groups like Dignity to suggest that homosexuality was not a sin: perhaps, maybe, it was a gift from God. And if that were the case, why ban the natural expression of that gift?

The Ratzinger letter sought to quash that line of thinking.

"Although the particular inclination of the homosexual person is not a sin," the 1986 letter argued, "it is a more or less strong tendency ordered toward an intrinsic moral evil; and thus the inclination itself must be seen as an objective disorder."

Put another way: Love the sinner, sure, but remember, this particular sinner's very identity is objectively disordered.

The Halloween letter specifically addressed Catholics who believed gay sex could be moral: "It is not." Not only was it immoral, but a sexually active gay person was declared "essentially self-indulgent." The letter never explicitly addressed the AIDS crisis, but it did make an oblique reference, stating that the "practice of homosexuality may seriously threaten the lives and well-being of a large number of people." The "gay plague" language bandied about in the White House briefing room seemed now to find its way to Rome.

Defenders of the letter pointed out that it also prohibited gay bashing, a growing threat as more people were honest about their sexual orientation. Several US bishops had preached against this kind of violence, including Cardinal Joseph Bernardin in Chicago and Cardinal John O'Connor in New York. The Halloween letter echoed those calls. "It is deplorable that homosexual persons have been and are the object of violent malice in speech or in action," it read. "Such treatment deserves condemnation from the Church's pastors wherever it occurs."

But the church's denunciation of gay bashing, the letter stated, should not give people license to claim "the homosexual condition is not disordered." And because of that disorder, gay people who were vocal about their orientation and practices might prompt "irrational and violent reactions" from others.

That is, gay bashing is wrong, but gays shouldn't be surprised when it happens.

Why was the church making life so difficult for gay men—especially during such a terrifying time? The letter infuriated David Pais. Father Bill was heartbroken. Gay Catholics were outraged. "Not being surprised at violence directed against gays and lesbians is tantamount to saying that fag-bashing is OK, as un-Christianlike, as un-Christlike, as hateful a thing as a Church can say," Dignity raged in an editorial.

But the group urged its members to stay and fight for their faith. "We Catholic lesbians and gay men are as much the Church as Pope John Paul II and the hierarchy," the essay continued. "We can affect the Church by making our presence and views known."

———

Following the expulsion from Saint Francis Xavier, David Pais and other members of Dignity eventually found a home at an Episcopal church where they met for Mass. But it wasn't the same. David was angry.

"When we were asked to leave the parish, I felt like I was being thrown out of my home," he told me.

Though he felt beaten down, David had a little bit of fight left in him. He loved the community at Saint Francis Xavier, and he felt it was worth trying to salvage. He joined a protest movement called the Cathedral Project, in which members of Dignity New York attended Mass at Saint Patrick's Cathedral, the home church of Cardinal O'Connor. They weren't there to make worshippers uncomfortable. They sat quietly in their pews and participated in Mass.

But when the priest began to preach, members of the group stood and turned their backs to the altar. "We were acting as witnesses to the refusal of the church to love all of its members equally," David said. But, he added, "we really didn't want to disrupt the Mass. At least, I didn't want to disrupt the Mass. Because for me, I respected why people were there. I just really wanted to say, we have a right to be here too. We have a right to be welcomed into this house of God."

The protests continued for several months, but they didn't seem to be working. Cardinal O'Connor stood firm in his decision to evict Dignity. But he wanted the protests to cease, so the archdiocese filed lawsuits and called police. Some of the protesters were arrested inside the church when they refused to sit down. David took all the confrontation to heart.

He had lost dozens of friends to AIDS and was dealing with his own HIV diagnosis. Then he had been told he was intrinsically disordered and was booted out of his church. He decided he was fed up. He had to leave the church.

"I distinctly stepped away," he recalled. "'Bolted' might be a better term."

The rationale was self-evident: "I can't spend all my time and energy being angry and fighting the church—not when I need it for survival."

He was done with his faith. For now.

7

SAINT VINCENT'S

Smack dab in the middle of Greenwich Village, Saint Vincent's Hospital has a history as colorful as the generations of women who staffed its wards, the Sisters of Charity of New York. In the hospital's first year, 1849, cholera plagued New York, and Saint Vincent's responded, providing medical care to the working-class Irish immigrants who lived in nearby tenements. Decades later, when the *Titanic* sank, in 1912, rescuers pulled terrified survivors from the icy waters and eventually transported them to Saint Vincent's. Nearly a century after that disaster, the proximity of the hospital to the World Trade Center meant that it became a hub serving victims of 9/11. But perhaps the tragedy most associated with Saint Vincent's Hospital occurred in the 1980s and '90s, when its doctors, nurses, and chaplains responded to the HIV and AIDS crisis with surprising alacrity, transforming a 130-year-old Catholic hospital into a refuge for gay men.

Given its history, I sought to learn all I could about this hospital. But it wouldn't be easy. Whereas I could visit Saint Veronica's to see the

AIDS memorial and Saint Francis Xavier to stand in the sanctuary where Dignity held its defiant Mass, Saint Vincent's closed in 2010. The closure was the result of years of mismanagement, a changing healthcare landscape, the financial cost of the hospital's commitment to care for the poor, or a combination thereof. No one seems to agree.

That more recent history was not my primary concern. I instead was focused on a relatively short period in the life of the hospital, the 1980s and '90s. I dug through newspaper archives, searching for insight into how Saint Vincent's became nearly synonymous with AIDS. From there, I tracked down doctors, nurses, priests, nuns, and volunteers who worked with people with AIDS at the hospital. I asked them to paint a picture of the daily rhythm of the place. That helped, but I still didn't feel like I grasped its full significance. So finally, I decided to make a visit to the site of the former hospital, to see if I could feel something by standing there, closing my eyes and taking in what many people had told me was hallowed ground.

Because I'm only in New York occasionally, and for a few days at a time, I decided to make something of a pilgrimage out of my visit. I took the subway to Chelsea and then walked a few blocks to Saint Francis Xavier. I spent several minutes inside, reflecting on David's poignant observation that this church was where countless numbers of gay men prayed for strength and healing during the height of the AIDS crisis. I thought about Father Bill celebrating Mass here, and how his ministry reached people in need of spiritual solace. Trying to clear my mind, I stood in front of the carved statue of Saint Aloysius Gonzaga. With my head now in the right space, I left the church for my trek to the old Saint Vincent's.

It was a warm, late afternoon in the waning days of summer. The stroll let me avoid the hustle and bustle of a rush-hour subway ride and gave me time to continue meditating. Plus the route I had planned would take me past places that are now LGBT landmarks. I headed to the

Stonewall Inn, the iconic gay bar that is home to the start of the modern gay rights movement, for a beer with a couple of friends. From there, I walked a few more blocks and suddenly found myself at the site of the old hospital, many of its buildings refurbished and converted into luxury residences.

Several images from the hospital grounds caught my attention. Still standing are the elaborately carved door frames, one with a caduceus, the staff with a snake curling around it, the symbol of medicine. Below it, in all capital letters, "St. Vincent's Hospital." Another doorway, this one beige concrete set against red brick, includes a three-dimensional likeness of a Sister of Charity, wearing a nurse's bonnet and keeping watch over the entryway.

Across the way, in a small sliver of green space boxed in by three busy streets, sits a park that serves as a memorial to the former hospital. A series of markers are inlaid around the perimeter of the red paver–lined walkway, each one the size of a manhole cover, marking historical moments in the life of Saint Vincent's.

"Former Site of Saint Vincent's Hospital 1849–2010" reads one in all capital letters. "The Sisters of Charity founded the hospital to care for the poor and disadvantaged." I walk from marker to marker, searching for the medallion that commemorates the AIDS crisis. I find it and snap a photo. A folded piece of ribbon sits in the middle, a carved depiction of the red lapel accessory that a graduate of a Catholic high school had created in 1991 to draw attention to AIDS. It reads, "Saint Vincent's opened the first and largest AIDS ward on the East Coast in 1984." A man sees me looking around and approaches, introducing himself as a local historian. After he learns what I'm looking for, he recalls the dark days when gaunt, frail young men walked these very streets. I ask about the nuns who ran the hospital and he takes a breath.

"The only people to stay behind and take care of the dying and the sick," he says, "were the Sisters of Charity, following their Christian mission."

I decide to sit down on one of the benches as the area around me grows hectic. Commuters cut through the park, rushing to the subway. A young couple embraces, seemingly oblivious to the honking horns and distracted pedestrians. The sun begins to set. I spend a few more minutes contemplating the scene around me, trying to block out the chain stores that have displaced smaller, independent businesses and pushing away thoughts about the hospital having been chopped up and developed into expensive condos. Instead I imagine these grounds as they were back then, home to a place where so many young gay men spent their final days. Where their boyfriends and families, biological and chosen, fed them meals, read them stories, and quietly prayed for deliverance from the pain and anguish. I take a deep breath and wonder again how this had come to pass. With the sun now set, I join the throngs of people walking by these buildings, now in a hurry to get somewhere else.

———

The story of how Saint Vincent's Hospital came to provide a refuge for gay men dying from AIDS is more complicated than I first imagined. A Catholic hospital in the 1980s didn't transform overnight into a place where gay men felt comfortable during particularly vulnerable moments. In the end, many received excellent medical care, and eventually the hospital treated them better than many other parts of society had. But that reality required time and effort. It took Catholic nuns who were committed to learning how to serve this particular community and queer activists who refused to settle for less than what they deserved. The give and take between these two seemingly at-odds groups resulted in what would become one of the finest AIDS clinics anywhere in the United States. Part of the transformation, I learned, was due to the tenacity of the medical staff, including a young doctor who was a rising star in HIV and AIDS medicine, as well as a group of nuns who weren't afraid to admit when they needed help living up to their ideals.

Dr. Ramon Torres, who goes by Gabriel, led the AIDS clinic at Saint Vincent's for about a decade, but his history with the hospital stretches back even longer. When he took the job, he was a young startup in the new field of HIV and AIDS medicine, one of many gay doctors who stepped up to care for their community. Dr. Torres knew the Catholic Church was conservative when it came to homosexuality, but he nonetheless admired its outreach to the poor and undocumented.

"The archdiocese opened their arms basically to those groups that have been neglected by other providers of care," he recalled thinking as he weighed the job offer.

Though he anticipated there might be challenges practicing HIV and AIDS medicine at a Catholic institution, he accepted the job and got to work.

Dr. Torres wanted to begin his tenure at Saint Vincent's with a gesture of goodwill. The clinic was located in an auxiliary building that stood apart from the main campus, so it had something of an independent feel. That distance enabled him to provide the kind of care he deemed necessary, regardless of church teaching on sexuality. Still, he wanted the hospital administrators to know he appreciated their commitment to men with HIV and AIDS who couldn't afford medical care anywhere else. He found a religious goods catalog and ordered a cross. When it arrived, he hung it by the clinic's entrance, hoping to connect the clinic visually to the hospital, where crosses hung in hallways and patient rooms. That's when Dr. Torres's pager beeped. The president of the hospital wanted to talk.

The hospital had strict guidelines when it came to religious iconography, Dr. Torres remembers being told. Like most Catholic institutions, Saint Vincent's displayed crucifixes, with the body of Jesus affixed to the cross. The bare cross in the clinic would have to be removed. Dr. Torres couldn't believe it. He was trying to build bridges to the hospital. Was he really being lectured about choosing the wrong kind of cross? It seemed ridiculous, but he did what he was told.

The story stuck with Dr. Torres even decades after he left Saint Vincent's. He told me it was a harbinger of future confrontations.

"I was allowed to stay there," he said, "but only under the condition that I follow the rules."

———

Before he entered AIDS care, Dr. Torres planned to work with vulnerable populations suffering from diabetes. But life got in the way of those plans. Dr. Torres grew up in Puerto Rico. He moved to New York in 1976 and enrolled at New York University, the first in his family to go to college. He graduated and started medical school at Columbia, signing up for a program that covered tuition in exchange for helping at-risk and underserved communities.

Then 1983 happened.

About 2,800 Americans were already diagnosed with AIDS by then, and nearly half of those cases were in New York. Saint Vincent's was doing what it could to help. Gabriel, as a medical student, was assigned to a visiting rotation at the hospital. He couldn't believe the illness he saw, especially among people of color.

"It was very shocking to see the devastation," he recalled of those first days at Saint Vincent's. "I mean young, robust, muscular gay men from the Village literally dying." In the emergency department, Gabriel encountered patients arriving very sick, carried in by friends, unable to stand or walk on their own. Their arms were covered in purple lesions. Some had them all over their necks and faces.

"All around the hospital," Gabriel recalled, "you saw Kaposi's sarcoma and vascular dermatosis, a growth that turns your skin violaceous—it looks like you have grapes growing out of your skin, pendulous grapes; I mean your body is covered entirely with it."

Those images, sounding like something taken from the pages of the Bible, shook Gabriel. He decided he wanted to help the community—his community. Saint Vincent's seemed like the place to do it. In 1987, a few years after his first rotation there, Gabriel accepted a job at the hospital, running a medical clinic for men who were homeless.

He threw himself into the emerging world of HIV and AIDS medicine. He saw the need for more information about this still little-understood disease, so he sought to learn as much as possible and then share it with the medical community. He launched a study of how AIDS affected the homeless population and presented the findings two years later. It caught the eyes of social workers and the media, and Dr. Torres was featured in an article that appeared on the front page of the metro section of the *New York Times*.

Dr. Torres found that the HIV infection rate at a single homeless shelter was a staggering 62 percent, far above the rate in the general population. The implication was clear: the city was failing its homeless residents. With his research, Dr. Torres brought a new understanding to how the disease made its way into vulnerable populations and with it, increased attention from the media. That was a good combination for a hospital seeking to carve out a place for itself in responding to HIV and AIDS. The following year, in 1990, Saint Vincent's asked Dr. Torres to lead its AIDS clinic.

Saint Vincent's AIDS clinic helped the institution live out its mission of serving the marginalized while simultaneously becoming a valuable source of income for the hospital. Dr. Torres encouraged patients to sign up for clinical trials at a time when pharmaceutical companies sought people willing to try experimental drugs. At one point, the hospital and the AIDS clinic received perhaps hundreds of millions of dollars a year because of these trials. At the same time, Dr. Torres was intent on making sure that vulnerable populations had access to quality care through the clinic, a goal supported by the Sisters of Charity of New York. This meant that in addition to serving the primarily gay men who lived nearby in Greenwich Village, the clinic made sure that people who were homeless, from all over the city, also received care. In addition, Saint Vincent's also focused on serving undocumented immigrants, young mothers and their babies, transgender people, and sex workers, populations all at higher risk of contracting HIV.

————

That commitment to the poor and marginalized was part of what made Saint Vincent's Hospital unique, but a culture of holistic care made it special. The hospital tried to celebrate life even in the midst of unrelenting death. Although the AIDS ward was never a cheery place, it wasn't a hopeless one either. Perhaps no one tried harder than Sister Patrice Murphy, who coordinated supportive care at the hospital's AIDS hospice. Sister Patrice attended trainings at the Gay Men's Health Crisis early on when she decided she wanted to help make life easier for gay men dying from AIDS. At Saint Vincent's, she supervised chaplains and patients. Sister Patrice radiated love, and she set the mood on the floor.

Patients were attracted to her sense of humor. Activists were encouraged by her open-mindedness. Chaplains were drawn in by her warmth. Father Bill McNichols met with Sister Patrice each morning, when she shared stories from the night before—like her visits to gay bars, where she accepted awards from activists. She found that so funny: a nun in a gay bar. Then she handed Father Bill a list of patients to visit that day. It was somber work, but Sister Patrice found joy in it, joy that inspired

Father Bill and the other volunteers. They couldn't help their patients with medicine, but they could try to be with them in difficult moments.

The volunteers on the AIDS wards loved one time of year in particular: Christmas, when they tried to lessen the gloominess on the floor with visits from Santa and Mrs. Claus—in drag. That is, a woman playing Santa and a man dressed up as Mrs. Claus. The Kringles handed out gifts and made silly jokes. They simply tried to make patients smile.

Then there were the nurses. Saint Vincent's had trained thousands of nurses, and Dr. Torres boasted that it had some of the best ones in the city. One nurse remembers a patient who was a classically trained pianist. He had gone to Juilliard, and her heart broke when she had to prick his hands with needles. He hated seeing the needle go in. The pain was too much. She wished she could tell him he could be discharged and that he could go back to playing. But there was hardly any good news like that in those early days.

Still, that nurse came to see her role on the AIDS ward as more than a job. Sister Patrice helped her connect her visits to patients to her Catholic faith. Sister Patrice explained the importance of kindness and mercy, even in an otherwise dreary hospital room. She showed the nurse one of Father Bill's drawings, depicting Jesus, covered in purple KS lesions. Sister Patrice encouraged the nurse to show small gestures of intimacy that made her patients feel human again. So the next time the nurse saw the pianist, she asked him how it felt to be able to create such beautiful music. His eyes lit up as he described how much he enjoyed sharing beauty with other people.

————

Dr. Torres eventually raised funds to expand the clinic, though he said he found it difficult to get the hospital to reinvest as much money as he thought was needed for it to thrive. Still, success brought more success and Saint Vincent's became known as one of the leading research centers in AIDS medicine, at one point overseeing forty clinical trials. Most of his patients seemed to be gay men of color, Dr. Torres observed, from particularly vulnerable New York communities. He was proud of the clinic's work, even when it was exhausting and emotionally draining. There were times when Dr. Torres tried to keep the peace between the biological families of his patients and their boyfriends, acting not just as a medical doctor but as something of a social worker and psychologist. Other patients even became friends, finding in Dr. Torres a trusted confidante, such as a closeted priest from Philadelphia who visited New York regularly, first to meet other gay men and then to receive AIDS treatment at the hospital.

The clinic's educational component, vital to protecting public health, proved complicated for Dr. Torres. Saint Vincent's Hospital was Catholic. This meant a special commitment to care for the poor, which had drawn Dr. Torres to the clinic in the first place. But it also meant, officially at least, that the discussion and distribution of condoms was prohibited, as the Catholic Church taught that the use of artificial birth control was a sin. But the "officially" in that sentence is key, because even at the highest levels of the US church, there was disagreement about how Catholics should engage in public health efforts. Debates among bishops, who set policy for the church and its institutions, usually stayed private. But in this instance, the disagreement about condoms and HIV spilled into the public realm, with the fate of programs like the AIDS clinic at Saint Vincent's in the hands of powerful prelates.

8

LETTER OF THE LAW

The archbishop of New York had something to say. So Cardinal John J. O'Connor did what powerful people do when they have something to say: he called a press conference. It would take place on Sunday morning, December 13, 1987, immediately following Mass. He would speak to reporters gathered near the altar inside his church, Saint Patrick's Cathedral. He would look the part. He would wear his miter, the triangulated headgear that signified he was a prince of the church. He would hold his crosier, a long rod reminiscent of a shepherd's staff. He would speak clearly and calmly.

That Cardinal O'Connor would hold a press conference was hardly remarkable. He had used the media effectively since his arrival in New York nearly four years earlier to spread the church's message. He was a regular in the city's tabloids. He appeared on television and radio, speaking to New Yorkers and the nation. He spoke out on social justice issues often, to defend the rights of workers or to condemn anti-Semitism. So holding a press conference after Mass inside Saint Patrick's was not unusual, but the intended audience was.

When Cardinal O'Connor wanted to say something about the city, he called his friend the mayor. When he wanted to say something about the country, he wrote President Reagan, who just a few months earlier had appointed him to the White House AIDS commission. When he had something to say to ordinary Catholics in the pews, he preached at Saint Patrick's or wrote a column in the archdiocese's newspaper. But the cardinal's intended audience that morning was composed of other bishops. Bishops tended not to communicate with one another through the press. If they had something to say to another bishop, they made phone calls or sent letters. Bishops did not like their disagreements to be made public. But Cardinal O'Connor felt the moral clarity of the church was at stake, and mere phone calls and letters wouldn't do. So he called a press conference.

Cardinal O'Connor told reporters that morning that he disagreed with a policy paper released earlier that month by the national body of Catholic bishops. The organization routinely drafted papers about pressing societal issues, such as nuclear weapons, healthcare, and poverty. In some ways, there was perhaps no issue more pressing in American life by 1987 than AIDS. By the end of that year, more than forty thousand Americans died from the disease. There was no vaccine and no cure. Americans largely did not know how to protect themselves. Being diagnosed with HIV was akin to a death sentence.

Catholic bishops had finally responded to the AIDS crisis that fall with "The Many Faces of AIDS," a letter designed to raise awareness about the disease, to encourage Catholics to react compassionately toward those who were suffering, and to offer the church's vast healthcare and education systems as resources in the fight to slow the spread. The major breakthrough, however—at least as far as headline writers were concerned—was that the bishops expressed an openness, however small, to the possibility that condoms might be a morally licit way to fight HIV. That year, US Surgeon General C. Everett Koop pleaded with doctors to promote the use of latex condoms to help slow the spread of HIV. With its seeming openness to mainstream public health guidance, "The Many Faces of AIDS" seemed to call into question the church's total ban on artificial birth control, which had been hotly debated ever since the Vatican reaffirmed its prohibition in the 1960s.

Cardinal O'Connor said he understood the gravity of the AIDS crisis. After all, he pointed out, he visited patients on the AIDS wards at Saint Clare's and Saint Vincent's. He had condemned violence against gays, and he had helped Mother Teresa open the AIDS hospice at Saint Veronica's. But he was steadfast when it came to the church's ban on condoms, even in the fight to slow HIV.

So in his statement to reporters, the cardinal called the release of the letter "a very grave mistake." He said Catholics in New York would not be permitted to teach that condoms were effective against HIV. And he said he wasn't alone in his views.

"I think what will happen is that all over the United States you will find bishops issuing statements similar to mine," he said.

The cardinal's press conference did what he intended for it to do: it put on notice the bloc of moderate and progressive bishops who drafted, approved, and promulgated "The Many Faces of AIDS." The institutional church must not waver in its opposition to condoms or homosexuality, Cardinal O'Connor said, even as HIV and AIDS continued their path of destruction.

One of the drafters of "The Many Faces of AIDS" was Cardinal Joseph Bernardin, the archbishop of Chicago and the de facto head of the US hierarchy's more progressive wing, which had held power over the bishops' conference for decades. Cardinal O'Connor represented a new style of bishop in the United States, one more in line with Pope John Paul II's conservative vision for the church. While the two cardinals had disagreed before, they had never butted heads in such a public manner.

The process of drafting "The Many Faces of AIDS" had begun about six months earlier, in June 1987. The National Conference of Catholic Bishops announced the creation of a special committee to examine the church's response to the crisis. The committee's work was to consider how the church's healthcare, education, and media ministries treated the issue of AIDS. By 1987, some bishops, including Cardinal Bernardin, had already released statements on the epidemic, but the national conference had yet to do so. Cardinal Bernardin, who served on the special committee, knew that crafting a compelling pastoral response at a time when the institutional church seemed intent on stymieing the gay rights movement would be difficult, but he wanted to contribute to what he recognized was a growing national emergency.

The committee members sought to answer a few key questions. What kind of public policy should the church be advocating around HIV and AIDS? What forms of education were appropriate for Catholics? How could the church contribute to the wider conversation about AIDS?

They sent a draft of the document to public health experts, including the Centers for Disease Control, the Catholic Health Association, and medical professionals who had worked in HIV and AIDS care. They consulted theologians to make sure the document was in line with church teaching. Three drafts later, and following a review by the conference's executive committee, they released the letter, on December 7, 1987. The bishops felt they had achieved their elusive goal of writing a letter that contained practical contributions in the fight against HIV and AIDS while also upholding traditional church teaching about sexuality and condoms.

Initial reaction to the letter was predictable. Conservative Catholics seized on the language about condoms. A representative from the National Catholic Coalition lashed out at gay men, saying the document "does not clearly say what is wrong with the main cause of AIDS, and that is homosexuality." Gay rights activists slammed bishops. One member of the Illinois Gay and Lesbian Task Force said he was "sick of the Catholic bishops and their sanctimonious, prissy attitude toward gay sex." Gay Catholics once again found themselves stuck somewhere in the middle.

A gay Catholic activist in Chicago saw in "The Many Faces of AIDS" a positive step toward compassion. "It's better than silence because silence equals death," he said, invoking the rallying cry of the controversial activist group ACT UP. "I think the bishops are trying to deal with this issue as best they can. If they hadn't included it," he said, referring to the portion about condoms, "it would have fallen on deaf ears."

What the bishops actually said in "The Many Faces of AIDS" more or less mirrored the prevailing ethos of US Catholicism in 1987. A substantial portion was devoted to the rights of the poor to receive medical care, which was already happening at some Catholic hospitals, such as Saint Vincent's. Another part highlighted the connection between economic inequity and risky behavior, such as drug use. There was an emphatic call for Catholic hospitals to open their doors to those most in need. Regarding sexual ethics, the document didn't stray from traditional church teaching, stating, "We call upon all people to live in accord with the authentic meaning of love and sexuality." To bishops, that meant "a monogamous, heterosexual relationship of lasting fidelity in marriage." The text actually condemned public health campaigns promoting safe sex, which the document said would compromise human sexuality, "making it 'safe' to be promiscuous."

A few paragraphs toward the end of the document seemed to be the source of Cardinal O'Connor's ire. Those sections stated that public health campaigns, "if grounded in the broader moral vision outlined above, could include accurate information about prophylactic devices or other practices proposed by some medical experts as potential means of preventing AIDS." In other words, the bishops would not object to efforts to save the lives of at-risk populations, even if that meant telling sexually active gay men that condoms could help protect them from HIV, a now-standard teaching in public health campaigns. Perhaps anticipating conservative opposition, like the concerns eventually raised by Cardinal O'Connor, the letter included a disclaimer: "We are not promoting the use of prophylactics, but merely providing information that is part of the factual picture."

As for people with HIV, the letter stated that they may even be morally obliged to use condoms if they were sexually active, as their use protected the common good by slowing the spread of the virus. In an addendum to the document specifically about Catholic healthcare, however, the document reiterated that Catholic hospitals should advocate chastity. But in the context of a specific relationship with patients, it was permissible to talk about practices advocated by public health officials.

Cardinal O'Connor's press conference was picked up in newspapers across the nation, with reporters intrigued by the battle brewing between conservative and moderate wings of the US hierarchy. For his part, Cardinal Bernardin responded to the backlash created by Cardinal O'Connor with a column in Chicago's Catholic newspaper. He wrote that he regretted "some of the interpretations" about "The Many Faces of AIDS" he had seen in the press, pinning his criticism not on his fellow cardinal, but on the media.

As Cardinal O'Connor predicted, other bishops were drawn into the public disagreement and two distinct sides emerged: those who supported the letter and those who thought the church should draw a harder line against condoms. It was a relatively rare public display of disunity. A handful of bishops condemned the document, including Cardinal Bernard Law of Boston and Archbishop Theodore McCarrick of Newark.

"We cannot approve or seem to approve the distribution of information regarding contraceptive devices and methods which might leave some to think that they could in good conscience ignore or contradict this teaching," Cardinal Law said in a joint statement with other New England bishops shortly after the letter was published.

Other bishops were equally candid in their defense of the letter, acknowledging the reality that condoms were part of the solution in fighting AIDS. Another member of the letter's drafting committee, Cincinnati Archbishop Daniel Pilarczyk, asked, "Are we going to talk about condoms and 'safe sex' practices when we teach about AIDS?" His answer was unequivocal. "Yes, we are, because they are part of the whole picture. There is no point in pretending such things do not exist." Archbishop Pilarczyk maintained the letter did not endorse the use of condoms more broadly, but he pointed out it was simply "good sense" to highlight reality during a particularly challenging time.

Other bishops took aim directly at Cardinal O'Connor, accusing him of damaging the church's reputation by going public with his criticism of the letter. "I regret very much that Cardinal O'Connor publicly took issue with the statement," Archbishop Rembert Weakland of Milwaukee said. "I think he did irreparable harm to all of us by doing that."

At the Vatican, Pope John Paul II initially tried to distance himself from the controversy brewing in the United States. He told reporters that he would not tell American bishops how to handle it—but, he added, they "should reflect" on the issue because they "know what the doctrine of the church in this area is. And they should find their own expression for that which is in accord with the universal doctrine of the church." Rome eventually got involved about six months after "The Many Faces of AIDS" was published. Cardinal Joseph Ratzinger, who two years earlier condemned homosexuality in the "Halloween Letter," wrote that he and Pope John Paul II were concerned about both the language about the use of condoms and the public division on display among US bishops.

"To seek a solution to the problem of infection by promoting the use of prophylactics would be to embark on a way not only insufficiently reliable from the technical point of view, but also and above all, unacceptable from the moral aspect," he wrote.

When bishops met the following June, they debated behind closed doors about how to handle the controversy. With the Vatican taking Cardinal O'Connor's side, Cardinal Bernardin realized he had lost. He nonetheless urged the bishops not to rescind "The Many Faces of AIDS." Instead, he asked the group to draft a new letter that would supplement the original, and the bishops agreed.

The new document, "Called to Compassion and Responsibility: A Response to the HIV/AIDS Crisis," was released in November 1989. It repeated many of the themes from "The Many Faces of AIDS," condemning discrimination against people with AIDS and urging the expansion of AIDS ministries. But the new document called the promotion of condoms to fight the spread of HIV "poor and inadequate advice," contradicting the advice of reputable public health officials.

The resolution of this conflict over condoms showed that the conservative wing of the church was ascendant. For gay Catholics who still bothered to pay attention to official church documents even after the trauma of the "Halloween Letter," the kerfuffle was another sign that their bishops were not receptive to their pleas for acceptance.

I was curious how the debate affected the work being undertaken in Catholic hospitals, places where issues of life and death were confronted daily, far away from the bright lights of television cameras. After all, it's unlikely that bishops thought they could influence private decisions made by gay men about using condoms. But perhaps the letter affected the kind of care Catholic hospitals provided people with HIV and AIDS?

It's tempting to think that if bishops barred the promotion and distribution of condoms, that was the end of the debate. Because the press often focused on church leaders, news reports gave the impression that their battles were representative of the church. That was an easy trap to fall into, even for me when I researched this book. Catholic cardinals and archbishops in the 1980s and 90s wielded vast communications operations and were often savvy about propagating their views. But the reality on the ground told a different story.

For answers, I turned to a soft-spoken Catholic nun who helped lead Saint Vincent's during the height of the AIDS crisis. When I asked her about the public battle between two factions of US bishops, she didn't remember either of the documents. She pointed me to several nurses and doctors, people who had labored in the trenches, who might recall the debate. Yet each of them looked at me, puzzled, when I asked the same question. They had been focused on providing quality medical care with limited resources, not on hierarchical bickering.

That's not to say that the fraught issue of condoms in Catholic hospitals didn't cause the occasional conflict. Like nearly every other topic in this book, it's just more complicated than I first thought.

———

On Labor Day in 1989, more than three hundred protesters stormed the waiting room of Saint Vincent's emergency department. They chanted. They made speeches. They demanded change.

As the hospital staff cleaned up after the protesters had left, something caught a security guard's eye. Hanging on the wall of the waiting area was an image of the risen Christ. Rather than a traditional crucifix, this version depicts Christ as fully alive. He is resplendent in robes and he holds his arms stretched outward, his hands pointing upward to heaven. On those hands, protesters had unfurled condoms. The security guard was disgusted by what he saw and wanted the nuns to press charges. But the sisters weren't so sure.

Sister Karen Helfenstein worked at Saint Vincent's first as a nurse, and by the time the protest happened, she was the vice president for mission. As part of the administrative team, she would be partly responsible for deciding how to respond to the vandalism. But first, she wanted answers, help in understanding the reality of the situation at Saint Vincent's. What caused the protesters to invade the emergency room in the first place?

Sister Karen felt like an orchestra leader, using a baton to make peace between church authorities and gay rights activists. Her regular conversations with the medical staff convinced her that they were professionals who knew how best to treat their patients. If doctors and nurses said that patients needed access to condoms, she took them at their word. But Sister Karen also recognized the reality of Saint Vincent's situation. If Cardinal O'Connor saw the hospital distributing condoms, the AIDS clinic could be in trouble.

At Saint Vincent's, the use of condoms wasn't a theological or philosophical debate. Lives were literally at stake. So Sister Karen sat with the archdiocese's theologians and ethicists, who listened while she explained the clinic's dilemma. She was persuasive. Eventually, she and the ethicists had achieved a sort of peace: doctors and nurses could distribute information about condoms, and patients could be directed to nearby pharmacies to buy them. The archdiocese wouldn't interfere.

But the compromise didn't work for Dr. Torres. Many of his patients in the clinic were homeless. They needed more than information; they needed free condoms. To him, it was truly a matter of justice. Yet he also knew that he would not win a battle with Cardinal O'Connor, so he had to get creative.

"Obviously, we broke the 'law,' and we gave condoms under the table, even though we knew that we were running the risk of severe repercussions."

Dr. Torres wasn't alone in this guerilla healthcare. Other doctors and nurses kept condoms hidden in their desks. Distributing them to patients was against the rules, but it was an open secret that it happened. Some medical staff referred to them jokingly as "the c-word."

"Over the years," Dr. Torres said, "there was more of a tolerance and more of a sort of bending of the rules. Not that we were openly displaying condoms in some bowl outside our clinic. But there was definitely less of an adherence to enforcing the rules."

When the nuns learned that condoms were being distributed, they often looked the other way. A truce seemed to be working. Hospital policy prohibited the distribution of condoms, which satisfied church authorities. But they were handed out anyway, which made Dr. Torres feel like he was doing everything he could to fight AIDS.

So why, then, the nuns wondered, did three hundred people feel compelled to protest in the waiting room? Why did someone put condoms on an image of Christ? What, exactly, was the message the protesters were trying to send? Sister Karen decided the best way forward was to do what she had done with the cardinal's office and with the medical staff. She would listen.

"We need to talk with them, and we need to see what we can do, learning from them what their needs are," Sister Karen decided.

————

The sisters met with the protest organizers, who were from the AIDS Coalition to Unleash Power, or ACT UP. The group had formed in 1987, two years before the action in the emergency room. Stories about harassment at the hospital had been circulating in the gay community.

"They're not letting in their lovers to see them," recalled Gerri Wells, a member of ACT UP. "Security guards were being abusive towards gay people getting in there."

One story in particular caught more attention than others.

For many LGBT New Yorkers, Labor Day weekend meant the return of Wigstock. For twelve hours, attendees sported dresses, walked in heels, and wore wigs. Thousands of people attended in 1989, including Darren Britton. Darren and his friends were in drag, having fun, when a small group of men approached. They were not wearing wigs or dresses or heels or elaborate makeup. They instead carried lacrosse sticks, which they quickly turned into weapons, beating Darren and his friends.

A gay man in drag approached the cops. He pointed at the lacrosse players and told the police what happened. The police at first ignored the lacrosse players, deciding instead to arrest the man in the dress. Others saw the brutality and yelled for the police to help. The police eventually rounded up the lacrosse players and summoned an ambulance. Darren had been badly hurt, with terrible pain in his shoulders. He was hoisted into the ambulance and was on his way to Saint Vincent's.

Darren checked in and was shown to an exam room. But before he saw a doctor, he left and walked back to the waiting area. He told his friend that he had been subjected to verbal abuse from some of the hospital staff. Someone had called him a faggot. They made fun of his wig and his dress.

Darren's friend tried to help by escorting him back to the exam room. If the staff were going to continue harassing Darren, at least now he would have an ally and advocate by his side. But a security guard stepped in. He put on a pair of gloves, presumably because he assumed that the men were gay and possibly HIV-positive, and told Darren's friend that he wasn't allowed into the exam room. Darren was furious, but he was also in pain and needed help. Rather than argue with the security guard, he said goodbye to his friend and walked back by himself. He told other gay friends about the experience, and a reporter in one of the city's gay magazines wrote a story, which is how ACT UP heard about the abuse.

When an ACT UP member raised the idea of protesting Saint Vincent's, Gerri was all in. Cardinal O'Connor regularly highlighted AIDS care at Saint Vincent's as an example of the church's good work in the fight against HIV. Gerri had been raised Catholic and she described

Saint Vincent's as "the cardinal's baby." A loud protest would catch the hospital's attention, Gerri figured, and both the cardinal and the hospital would have no choice but to respond. She was right. After the protesters put condoms on the cross, hospital administrators certainly took notice. But the response by Sister Karen and other hospital administrators was something of a surprise.

When the sisters and other administrators asked the protesters why they targeted the hospital, ACT UP members described various grievances. It was more than just the one Wigstock incident. ACT UP's members felt the guards were rude to gays and lesbians. Sometimes, the people in the waiting room weren't simply friends, but partners and lovers. They were chosen family. But they often weren't allowed into the exam rooms because they were not related by blood or by law. Someone could be going through the worst moment of his life, alone in an unfamiliar setting, and his partner was not allowed to be with him. On top of that, some of the physicians and nurses would crack an occasional homophobic joke, maybe something they heard on a late-night show, thinking they were out of earshot of patients. The protesters wanted to change the hospital's culture, to make the institution more welcoming of the community it served.

The negotiations took a while, but little by little, the protesters and the hospital made progress. Staff were ordered to undergo sensitivity training. They were reminded that part of the hospital's mission was to support people through difficult moments, regardless of their sexual orientation.

"People are simply grieving and helping each other through a terrible time in their lives," Sister Karen reminded her colleagues. Saint Vincent's never pressed charges in response to the desecration of the statue. Instead of going on the defensive, it changed and became a refuge for gay men. In no small part, that was because a group of nuns chose to listen to a community that refused to be silenced.

But ACT UP wasn't done protesting the church.

9

"STOP THE CHURCH"

New York City was bitterly cold two weeks before Christmas in 1989. Wind whipped down the street and the thermometer was stuck in the twenties. Sean Strub picked up the pace. He hadn't been to church in years, but he desperately wanted to get inside Saint Patrick's Cathedral. As he approached the church, he knew this would be no ordinary Mass. Thousands of people stood on Fifth Avenue. Screaming. Chanting. Cheering. Some of the protesters, mostly young men and women in their twenties, held signs. "Condoms Not Prayer!" splashed across one. "Cardinal O'Connor won't teach safe sex," read another. "Curb your dogma," a third. Some protesters threw condoms into the street, and a few taunted the cops on hand to keep the peace. Even Jesus was there—someone dressed in white robes and a crown of thorns. He yelled into a bullhorn, telling the church to live up to the ideals of its founder.

The weeks leading up to the protest at Saint Patrick's had been chaotic. With the success of their other actions fueling change, including at Saint Vincent's, ACT UP wanted to take on Cardinal O'Connor specifically. Each year since his arrival to New York, Cardinal O'Connor's actions angered gay activists. The archdiocese, under his direction, sued in 1984 to overturn a city ordinance that prohibited employment discrimination against gays. He blocked gay Catholics from protesting in front of the cathedral in 1985. He organized a campaign against a gay civil rights bill in 1986. He pressured the city into promoting abstinence instead of condoms in 1987. He refused to reconsider his ban on Dignity after gay Catholics protested in 1988. Now it was 1989, and nearly ninety thousand Americans were dead from AIDS. ACT UP was angry, and they wanted Cardinal O'Connor to know. As one member put it years later, the protest was "designed as a confrontation, a revolt, a rebellion, a resistance."

Despite all the mayhem, and his inclination to demonstrate, Sean Strub didn't have time to be distracted by the commotion outside the cathedral. He had to think. His boyfriend had died from AIDS one year ago, so today could be cathartic. But first he had to find a seat inside.

———

My earliest understanding of ACT UP was binary. On one side were the hip and mostly young activists who wore jeans and "Silence=Death" t-shirts, featuring the now iconic hot pink triangle. Think of the colorful street art of Keith Haring, who created several projects to raise money for ACT UP before his death from AIDS in 1990. Members of ACT UP, including Sean Strub, were angry that society didn't take AIDS seriously and they weren't afraid of making people uncomfortable to get the attention their community needed. That meant protesting the church and its leaders. On the other side were ordinary Catholics who bristled at ACT UP's extremism and in-your-face tactics.

There was no middle ground, at least in my limited understanding of the dynamic. And to be fair, my impressions weren't totally off. ACT UP harbored a bias against the Catholic Church because of its stance against homosexuality and condoms and also because of its opposition to abortion. Catholic leaders regularly denounced the group. Even Catholics who were sympathetic to ACT UP's cause thought some of the protesters unfairly targeted the church when so much of society failed to respond to AIDS. But two items complicated my understanding of the dynamic between ACT UP and the Catholic Church.

First, Father Bill McNichols told me he actually attended an early meeting of ACT UP. That this gentle priest was attracted to a rowdy activism group prompted many questions. What drew him in? As a priest, did he have any reservations attending the meeting? Did he think it was possible to be a faithful Catholic and a member of ACT UP? He understood the rage ACT UP felt toward various institutions, including the church. Similar feelings filled his heart at times. But Father Bill found their fierce tactics a bit too much. He preferred candlelight vigils over noisy protests. The first ACT UP meeting Father Bill attended was his last, but he empathized with the group's goals.

Later, I read about a study that found about a third of the people who belonged to ACT UP were raised Catholic. That's higher than the Church's share of the general US population in 1989, when about 22 percent of Americans were Catholic. Most ACT UP members who had been raised Catholic had left the church, but about 7 percent of the respondents to the survey were still practicing. That meant the decision to protest Saint Vincent's and Cardinal O'Connor was supported by at least some practicing Catholics. In a way, the findings weren't entirely surprising. Cities in which ACT UP took to the streets, New York especially, were home to large Catholic populations. So in some ways, ACT UP chapters simply mirrored their cities. Still, the fact that some Catholics attended Mass on the weekend and ACT UP meetings during the week challenged what I increasingly understood to be my ignorant understanding of the group. I needed someone to help me grasp the dynamic. That's what led me to Sean Strub.

Sean was born into a large Catholic family in Iowa. His parents had named each of his three sisters Mary. Around age twelve, Sean started to feel that something about him was different. He couldn't pinpoint it, but he knew he was not like other boys. He sensed that it was a problem, however, and thought he had found a solution: the priesthood. Sean's father revered the church and it just made sense to him that whatever was wrong could be fixed by becoming a priest. Sean eventually accepted that he was gay, and then he grew disillusioned with Catholicism. To Sean, staying Catholic felt damaging, so he walked away.

In the 1980s, Sean was consumed with HIV and AIDS and how the virus spread relentlessly through his community. He was tested in 1985 and waited two agonizing weeks for the results, every moment filled with fear and anxiety about his future. If there was a future at all. Not sure what else to do, Sean turned to something he had long since left behind.

"I tried reciting the Catholic prayers of my childhood, something I hadn't done in years," he recalled.

Sean was thrown into a daze when the test came back positive. He had HIV. His partner, Michael, promised support and said he would be there for Sean, but reiterated that he did not want to be tested. For the next few years, Sean learned everything he could about HIV and devoted his fundraising and marketing skills to bringing awareness to the fight against AIDS.

Three years later, in November 1988, Sean's partner was admitted to the hospital and diagnosed with cryptococcal meningitis. Another test confirmed what Sean and Michael had long suspected, that he was also HIV-positive. Doctors at Saint Vincent's did what they could to bring Michael back from the brink, but he eventually slipped into unconsciousness and died in early December. A couple of weeks before Christmas, Sean received a note from Michael's mother, written "in careful Catholic-school penmanship with a shaky hand," thanking Sean for being Michael's "special friend" and for looking after her now deceased son. As Sean put it later, "No response to Michael's death consoled me as much as his mother's gentle recognition of our relationship."

As the months following Michael's death wore on, Sean channeled his grief into activism. The anger Sean felt toward institutions that tried to block public health measures that could have protected his partner grew inside him. It was a no-brainer when other members of ACT UP suggested the group protest at Saint Patrick's Cathedral. Still, there was some internal debate. Taking on the church was a provocative idea. Maybe ACT UP should stick to protesting the government, Wall Street, and pharmaceutical companies?

But Sean saw in Cardinal O'Connor an influential political figure trying to shape public policy, someone he believed was unqualified for such a role. He did not have medical or public health training, yet the cardinal served on the White House's AIDS commission. He used his influence to fight gay rights, oppose public health measures, and claim that condoms were ineffective in fighting AIDS. Sean and some other members of ACT UP who had been raised Catholic were fed up, and Cardinal O'Connor's actions sealed the deal. If the Catholics in the group wanted to take on the church, ACT UP wouldn't stop them. The various subcommittees in ACT UP, called affinity groups, created a plan. The protest, now dubbed "Stop the Church," was on.

Most of the protesters planned to remain outside the cathedral. Those who wished to enter the building would seek to blend in with the congregation, trading jeans and leather coats for their Sunday best. Once inside, they would engage in a silent die-in, throwing themselves onto the floor to symbolize the eighty-nine thousand Americans who had died from AIDS. Various ACT UP affinity groups planned other parts of the protest, operating as cells and keeping their unique plans secret. The entire operation would not be in jeopardy if one group failed to pull off its planned part of the protest, and limiting who knew what would reduce legal consequences when inevitable arrests were carried out.

Sean was part of the "Hail Marys" affinity group. During communion, members of the Hail Marys would approach the altar. They wouldn't say the customary "Amen" when presented with the consecrated host. Instead, they would reply with a political statement related to ACT UP's work, with each member creating their own message. Sean had so much emotion bottled up inside that he didn't know how to fit it all into one short sentence.

Organizers had sought to create a massive event with thousands of people on hand, so ACT UP used the press to reach out to would-be protesters, advertising in the *Village Voice* and placing stickers about the event throughout the city. The group partnered with Women's Health Action and Mobilization, which opposed the church's lobbying against abortion. ACT UP urged anyone with sympathies for gay men to come protest the church's "murderous AIDS policy."

When he got word of the protest, Cardinal O'Connor refused to keep silent. He instructed Catholics not to worry about the event and urged would-be Mass-goers to resist responding with violence. But just in case things got out of hand, the cardinal invited both uniformed and undercover police to attend Mass. And the mayor. In other words, Cardinal O'Connor seemed to be saying, *bring it on.*

The day of the protest, church officials cleared out the vast cathedral after the early morning service. Worshippers joining Cardinal O'Connor's Mass had their bags searched as they entered the building. At the same time, an ACT UP affinity group passed out paper booklets, disguised to look like official church bulletins, to people entering the church. But inside, the decoy bulletins contained subversive messages. "The intrusion of O'Connor and the church hierarchy into politics and public health guarantees that ALL people will suffer from the murderous policies of the church."

Sean finally walked into the massive cathedral. He didn't recognize any of his friends, each undercover in respectable church-going attire. Sean had chosen his own clothes strategically that morning as well, wearing a "Silence=Death" t-shirt under his button-down shirt and heavy winter coat. There was no way the police would take him for a protester. And there were so many police. Some patrolled outside, stopping the costumed protesters from going in. Others stood guard inside along the perimeter. Sean took a seat at the front of the cathedral.

It was Advent, just two weeks before Christmas. Cardinal O'Connor, dressed in purple robes, thanked the police for joining the Mass. He said he was aware that some protesters were inside the church, but he urged calm. Mass continued: the first reading, a sung psalm, the second reading, an alleluia, a selection from the gospel. Then it was time for the cardinal to deliver his homily.

I've listened to a recording of the homily from that Sunday. Cardinal O'Connor barely made it two minutes into his sermon before one of the ACT UP affinity groups jumped into action. Some members threw themselves onto the cold marble floor and began to yell. Others chained themselves to pews. Cardinal O'Connor tried to ignore the distraction and continue with the sermon, but it became impossible to ignore the chaos as more protesters joined in. He stopped preaching and suggested the congregation stand up, pray the rosary, and let police do their work. At this point in the recording, it feels like Cardinal O'Connor's plan might actually work. Maybe the protest had failed? But then someone blew a whistle and screamed, "O'Connor, you're killing us! You're killing us! Just stop it! Stop it!" Cops moved in and arrested the protester. The tape stops shortly after that.

Mass resumed, and the Hail Marys waited patiently for their part in the event, when they would shout protest phrases after receiving communion.

Worshippers exited their pews and processed to the front of the church to receive the Eucharist, the most solemn ritual in the Catholic faith. One protester, a young man who had been raised by Catholic parents in Long Island, reached the front of the line. The priest placed the host in his hands.

"The body of Christ," he said.

Normally, a person receiving the Eucharist would respond with a simple, "Amen." But this was a protest.

"Opposing safe-sex education is murder!" the protester shouted.

He then did the unthinkable: he crumbled up the host and threw it to the ground. An act of blasphemy, desecrating what Catholics believe to be the body of Christ. Several priests rushed over to pick up and consume the broken host and cops arrested the protester. Communion continued.

Soon Sean walked to the front of the church. He was fairly oblivious to all the commotion near the desecrated host. He had seen some activity near the communion line but wasn't sure what exactly was happening. He still didn't know what he would say to the priest when it was his turn to receive communion. This was the height of his participation in the protest, so he had to think of something. And it had to be meaningful.

Sean removed his winter coat and left it in the pew before taking his place in line. As he approached the front, he unbuttoned his outer shirt, revealing the "Silence=Death" t-shirt. It was clear he was with ACT UP. Before he knew it, Sean was next in line.

"The body of Christ."

Pain that had welled up for so long rushed to Sean's throat. He was angry at everyone who had turned their backs on his partner. On him. On their community. Rage overtook him, and Sean said his response clearly and loudly.

"May the Lord bless the man I love, who died a year ago this week."

The man I love. The words echoed in Sean's ears. The priest didn't hesitate or pull back his hands. He didn't ask Sean to leave. He handed him the host. Sean did just as he had countless times as a child growing up

Catholic in Iowa: he consumed the Eucharist. When he returned to his seat, he thought of his partner. That had been the first time he ever vocalized the words "the man I love" to another person. It was inside a church, a building that conjured up many emotions for Sean. The rest of the day would be a blur.

————

When Sean and I speak on the phone in 2020, I have trouble hearing him. A GPS blares directions in the background. He tells me that he and his partner are driving from Pennsylvania to visit Sean's father in Iowa. He says he has plenty of time to talk, but that I might have to put up with some background noise. Suddenly, I hear a blaring siren. Sean stops speaking for just a second, then apologizes again.

"One residual little piece of the Catholic faith sort of sticks with me," he explains. "I can't hear an ambulance without saying a two-second prayer in my head." He laughs. "Not the worst habit."

With the sirens gone, I ask Sean his thoughts on the church today. He repeats a theme I hear from other gay activists who grew up Catholic and have since walked away from the church.

"I worked early on at shedding what to me felt like the damaging parts of Catholicism," he says. He pauses, perhaps not content to leave it there. "But there are other parts of Catholicism that I embraced." His lifetime devotion to activism and social justice causes was not coincidental. "It really came out of that exposure to the church."

I think about how much the church lost by pushing out people like Sean. How much richer the church would be if its leaders had taken a deep breath, stopped talking, and listened.

————

While it's likely that at least some of the protesters were motivated by anti-Catholic bias, for many of them, including Sean, the event was meant to call attention to the church's efforts to shape public health policy. By opposing the use of condoms to fight HIV, some Catholic leaders, including Cardinal O'Connor, went against the advice of medical doctors who believed gay men and others at risk of infection needed unfiltered information. One of those doctors was a young Anthony Fauci. I talked to him on the phone about another pandemic, decades later, which would kill hundreds of thousands of Americans. But I knew that he had been an instrumental public health physician during the height of HIV and AIDS, so I asked what he thought of the church's public role during that time.

Dr. Fauci had been raised by his Catholic parents not to look down on anyone and to step up to help whenever he could. Those lessons were fortified by his teachers and professors at his Jesuit high school and college, he told me, but he didn't agree with the hardline positions he heard later as an adult from Catholic leaders against rights for women, gays, and people who might not fit neatly into the categories they seemed to believe were essential to a moral life.

The Jesuit commitment to intellectual honesty impressed Dr. Fauci when he was a student. By the time he took over the National Institute of Allergy and Infectious Diseases in 1984, those lessons guided him to the realization that he needed to listen to the community being most affected by this new epidemic: gay men.

"When you're dealing with a disease, the people who are suffering most from the community, you've got to listen to what it is that they have to say about their experiences," he told me.

Dr. Fauci eventually understood that meant engaging in dialogue with gay activists, sex workers, and drug users. It took some prodding. Some gay activists, including some of the founders of the Gay Men's Health Crisis and ACT UP, accused him of not acting quickly enough to stop the spread of HIV. Others took him to task for not supporting the rights of people with AIDS to access experimental drugs. Dr. Fauci listened to their concerns, made adjustments, and eventually won their support.

As for the church, its messages seemed less concerned about promoting effective public health than about passing judgment on the kinds of people who were getting sick, he said.

"Certain elements of the church were not as accepting of the community who were afflicted because of the fact that it was predominantly a gay community, injection drug users, commercial sex workers," he recalled. "They were not as embracing of the people who were affected as they should have been."

As doctors and other public health officials realized condoms would help protect gay men from contracting HIV, Dr. Fauci couldn't believe what he was hearing from some bishops, including Cardinal O'Connor.

"He didn't show a degree of empathy or flexibility toward the gay community and what their needs were, what they were suffering from," he remembers thinking. "He was very, I think, rigid in his approach to them."

Dr. Fauci also faulted the church for spreading false information, including messages that flew in the face of everything public health experts knew about slowing the spread. Some high-profile bishops said that condoms might actually hurt those who used them. In 1987, the Archdiocese of Boston filmed television commercials about HIV and AIDS, but the ads frustrated public health experts with their suggestion that condoms were ineffective in fighting the spread of HIV. Then there was the more belligerent Catholic League for Religious Liberty and Civil Rights, which backed an ad campaign in 1994 on mass transit in New York, Boston, and Washington. "CONDOMS DON'T SAVE LIVES," read one ad. "But restraint does."

Dr. Fauci found that kind of dishonesty reprehensible and "completely out of line." Intolerance from some bishops grated on him, at odds with the message he had learned from his parents and the Jesuits about the importance of serving other people.

He eventually stepped back from the church, no longer practicing his faith regularly. Still, he credits the Jesuits with instilling in him an intellectual honesty and a sense of compassion for the marginalized and he has supported Catholic immigration and educational ministries. He wonders how history might have looked had more church leaders lived out those values in the public square.

As he imagines it, "A lot of lives would have been saved."

———

As for Cardinal O'Connor, the protest didn't seem to affect his public standing. City and state politicians, even some with whom he clashed regularly, came to his defense. About a month after the protest, the cardinal was back in the news. Two men had viciously stabbed a gay Catholic man to death on Staten Island, the attackers hurling anti-gay invective. Cardinal O'Connor presided at the funeral Mass and even came around to endorse a hate crimes law that included sexual orientation as a protected category. On the AIDS front, he announced that the archdiocese planned to spend another $15 million on AIDS healthcare. And he pledged to visit a perplexingly exact number of patients with AIDS in the city's Catholic hospitals: one thousand. (He later said during a TV interview that he had visited 1,100.)

Stories like this add to Cardinal O'Connor's complexity. They support the criticism from gay rights activists that he only showed compassion to gay men when they were dying. Yet many people I interviewed talked about the cardinal's warmth and pastoral sense—including Father Bill McNichols. When I asked him about Cardinal O'Connor, Father Bill told me he actually felt bad for him. After his talk was canceled in Scranton in 1987 and the organizers told him that someone from the bishop's office had intervened, Father Bill scheduled a meeting with the cardinal to find out what had transpired.

The day of the meeting, Father Bill was at ease. The room in the cardinal's residence was imposing, but he was confident in what he had to say. He was immediately made comfortable by Cardinal O'Connor's friendliness. So Father Bill got right to it.

"Did you tell people they couldn't come hear me speak in Scranton?"

The cardinal looked confused.

"No," he said. "I don't know anything about that."

Father Bill explained what had happened, how participants had been shut out from learning valuable information that might have eased the burdens of people suffering with HIV and AIDS.

"I'm sorry to hear that," the cardinal told Father Bill.

The meeting didn't last much longer, and Father Bill didn't find out who had actually caused the Scranton conference to be canceled. Cardinal O'Connor walked Bill to the door. He seemed to know a bit about Father Bill's AIDS ministry.

"I love that you're doing what you're doing," the cardinal told the young Jesuit.

Father Bill was touched by these words of encouragement. He knew that Cardinal O'Connor had angered the gay community. The cardinal said things about gay people that Father Bill disagreed with to his core. But as Father Bill looked around the capacious residence, he suddenly felt sorry for Cardinal O'Connor.

"If you were my age, I think you'd be doing exactly the same thing," he said as he walked through the tall doors.

As Father Bill made his way deep into bustling midtown, he looked back, the doors growing smaller and smaller with each step. The cardinal, watching Father Bill, waved and went inside, hidden within an institution causing so much pain for gay and lesbian people.

"My God, this man is a prisoner," Father Bill thought.

10

"YOU COULDN'T
SAY IT WAS WRONG"

Sister Carol couldn't believe the view. It was 1987 and she had just landed in New York. A sister who lived at the convent she and Mary Ellen would call home for the next few months picked them up from the airport. As the nuns drove over the Fifty-Ninth-Street Bridge the enormity of Sister Carol's decisions hit her. She had never even visited New York City. Yet here she was, with all of Manhattan on display to greet her. She looked, wide-eyed, at Sister Mary Ellen, her mind racing.

"Everything is just huge and big and amazing and coming at you like, oh my God," she thought.

Just a few years before, Sister Carol had turned forty and experienced something of a vocational crisis. She was burnt out from her intense nursing career and knew she needed a change. That change had been taking on homecare nursing in Belleville. And now, all of a sudden, here she was in New York, ready to learn all she could about gay life and AIDS care. It was heady stuff—had she the time to dwell on it. But the car pulled to a stop in Hell's Kitchen.

"Welcome to Sacred Heart Convent!" their driver said cheerfully.

Sister Carol was stunned by her surroundings. Garbage bags were piled high on the sidewalk, and the stench took her breath away. People were lying in doorways. And there was so much graffiti. Sister Carol thought she had seen poverty and urban decay back in the Midwest, in Detroit and St. Louis, but this was next-level. New York City in the 1980s was tough. Murder rates soared each year, and cheap drugs flooded the city. Muggings were common occurrences on the city's poorly maintained subways. Sensing Sister Carol's discomfort, one of the New York nuns offered a short introduction and some rules of the road.

"Number one, don't walk too close to the alley, because somebody will probably jump out and stab you," the sister explained calmly. "Number two, don't walk too close to a building, because an air conditioner will probably fall on you. And number three, don't carry a purse. You're gonna be here for six months, so you'll probably be mugged."

"Well, OK then," Sister Carol said.

The next morning, Sister Carol and Sister Mary Ellen would head to Saint Vincent's Hospital to meet some of the staff and the pastoral care team members. They would meet the chaplains, people like Father Bill McNichols, and learn about the kind of care people with AIDS received at the hospital. Sister Carol was excited by the possibilities of this new ministry, but she had much to learn.

When it was time to head out, she and Sister Mary Ellen realized they had no idea how to use the subway. They wound up getting off the train too early and became confused. But one thing was clear: they did not see a hospital.

They tried asking for directions but, recalling the warning they received back at the convent, they worried someone might try to rob or stab them. Plus, there were those dangerous air conditioners. They decided to walk.

And walk. And walk. They finally found the hospital, but they were sweating and tired and unsure where they had even been. Learning to navigate New York would take time. And the confusion on the subway was just the beginning.

One evening, Sister Carol walked home from Saint Vincent's, eager to clear her head after witnessing so much suffering on the AIDS floor. Not far from the convent, she thought she felt something on the back of her ankle-length skirt. She turned and saw a man lifting up her skirt. She reacted quickly, swatting at him with her folded-up copy of the *Times*. The man ran away, but Sister Carol was mortified. She made eye contact with a cop standing nearby, hoping he'd jump into action. He shrugged.

"I could arrest you for assaulting that guy!" the cop said, laughing uproariously.

"So this is New York," Carol thought.

While city life took some getting used to, the purpose of the visit was to learn about the services offered in New York for people at risk of contracting HIV. Sister Carol and Sister Mary Ellen stayed focused on that. Similar to what Sister Patrice and Father Bill had done when they wanted to learn about HIV and AIDS, Sister Carol and Sister Mary Ellen signed up for training at the Gay Men's Health Crisis, the group David Pais helped grow, so they could volunteer on an AIDS hotline at Saint Clare's Hospital.

Following the training, the two nuns got to work. The hotline was housed in a small office inside the hospital, with room for just a couple of phones, a table, and two chairs. There was a massive binder for Sister Carol to read that would acquaint her with some of the questions she might be asked by the callers, who phoned anonymously so they could ask candid questions about HIV and AIDS. The callers didn't know a middle-aged nun was on the other end of the phone. And they didn't hold back.

"Are threesomes more dangerous than sex with one guy?"

"Do all condoms work the same or are some better than others?"

"What about sex toys, are those safe?"

"I'm seventy-six years old, I've been married to my wife for more than fifty years, and I'm gay," one caller asked Carol. "How do I come out?"

How was a Catholic nun supposed to know?

"Please hold," Carol said, yelling over to her colleague for advice.

Sister Carol's visits to the city's AIDS wards didn't feel any more successful than her early efforts on the hotline. When she arrived at a patient's room one day, she found his empty bed. The patient was in the bathroom, so Carol sat down and waited for him to return. On a side table there was an issue of *Better Homes and Gardens*, so she picked it up and started reading.

But as she flipped through the pages, her jaw dropped. *Better Homes and Gardens*, she quickly realized, was just a shell. The hotline questions, however graphic, did not prepare her for what she saw tucked in the magazine: tips for better gay sex—with photo illustrations.

When the patient returned, he saw a middle-aged nun reading his magazine. Sister Carol looked at him sheepishly. She tried breaking the ice.

"Do you . . . do this kind of stuff?" she asked.

"Yeah," he said. He was unabashed. After all, it was Sister Carol who had read his magazine. Why should he feel embarrassed? "Does it make a difference?"

Sister Carol felt she owed her patients honesty, even if that meant admitting her uneasiness about a lifestyle she didn't understand.

"I really don't know," she said.

What Sister Carol didn't know was if she was capable of providing compassionate care to a community whose lives were so different from her own, who inhabited realities that appeared to run contrary to the teachings of the Catholic Church, the institution to which she had devoted her entire life. Sometimes it was all too much for her. She wasn't totally comfortable with hearing so much about sex. After a stint working the hotline, with the deluge of sex questions continuing unabated, Sister Carol went for a long walk to think and pray. When she returned to the convent, she vented to Sister Mary Ellen.

"I've had it up to here with sex," she said, holding her hand high above her head, her voice tinged with frustration. She considered packing up. She had given her big city adventure the college try, but it wasn't working out. Maybe she could do something else back in Belleville.

But Sister Mary Ellen reminded Sister Carol that she wasn't one to give up. She was a tough, Polish nun who didn't shirk responsibility. She just needed to give it a bit more time. Carol knew Mary Ellen was right.

The two sisters visited various clinics and hospitals around the city, which is how they met Will Wake, a nurse on one of the city's AIDS wards. Will was a lifelong Catholic who took a liking to the pair of Midwestern nuns. They reminded him of his own family. He appreciated that they were eager to learn, and he saw their kindness as authentic. They weren't as brassy as the New Yorkers he encountered all day. Plus there was a local connection: Will's dad had been stationed in Belleville when he was in the Air Force. It almost seemed fated that the three of them would hit it off. Will wanted the two nuns to be successful in their quest to learn more about HIV and AIDS and he knew just the person who could help.

Will's partner, Jim D'Eramo, was something of an expert when it came to HIV. He was a journalist who helped chronicle AIDS by keeping his readers up to date on the latest scientific research. Like Will, Jim was a lifelong Catholic with a soft spot for nuns. Will and Jim had met as volunteers at the Gay Men's Health Crisis, and they were eager to talk with anyone who wanted to contribute to the cause. Especially two Midwestern nuns. Perhaps over drinks in one of New York's gay bars.

Sister Carol was transfixed by Will and Jim. She felt safe asking them questions about the AIDS hotline, and she was comfortable being vulnerable around them. She told them she felt confused about everything she was learning. Jim was blunt, which at first took Sister Carol some getting used to, but it was a trait she eventually came to admire. Jim knew that for the disease to slow, people had to use technical language about how it spread from person to person. There could be nothing mealy-mouthed when it came to prevention. She listened and began to understand why the hotline questions were so graphic. The callers weren't trying to shock her; they were trying to save their lives.

During one of their group dinners, Sister Carol talked about her uncertainty about her work when Jim interrupted her. As I learned during my own interview with Jim, he's not shy about cutting through the noise and saying what's on his mind.

"Before you go anywhere trying to help a person with AIDS, you have to do two things," Jim told Carol. "You have to look at your own prejudices and biases, and you have to look at your own stand on sexuality. Otherwise you'll never get past your own hang-ups and understand what it means to be diagnosed with AIDS."

Jim's piece of advice made everything click for Sister Carol in a way that had so far been elusive. What he said made sense to her. The magazine with provocative photos of gay men and hotline questions about the risks of certain sex acts weren't the problem. The issues were Sister Carol's, and she had to deal with them if she wanted to be an effective ally in the fight against AIDS. That insight from Jim, the idea that Sister Carol needed to name her own biases before engaging in HIV and AIDS care, changed how she approached the rest of her time in New York. She saw her work in a new light. The shift in focus played a critical role over the next several weeks and gave her the ability to allow a chance meeting with a gay man outside the convent to change her life.

———

Through volunteering at Saint Clare's, Mary Ellen had met a man in his thirties named Robert. Despite their three-decades-wide age difference, the Midwestern nun and the gay New Yorker hit it off. Robert volunteered at the hospital because his partner, Josh, had AIDS. He thought helping others cope was the best way he could respond to the confusion caused by the diagnosis. Recognizing how well Sister Carol had responded to Will and Jim, Sister Mary Ellen introduced her to Robert as well, trying to put another face to the community being most affected by HIV.

One evening after dinner, Sister Carol stepped out of the convent for some air. As she sat on the stoop, she noticed Robert walking toward her. He seemed to be shaking. As he got closer, Sister Carol saw him crying uncontrollably, his hands trembling.

"Oh, Robert," Sister Carol said.

"Hi, sister," he replied through his tears.

Carol was quiet.

"Josh is dying and there is nothing I can do."

Sister Carol couldn't think of anything to say that would be helpful at that moment. So she did what she would do for any other person who was upset because a loved one was dying. She held Robert and let him cry into her shoulder. He eventually composed himself, thanked Sister Carol, and walked on. The next morning, Sister Carol learned that Josh had died overnight.

That moment stuck with Carol. She might never be comfortable with all the sex. After all, it was so different from her own life experience. But holding Robert, seeing how upset he was that Josh lay dying and that he was powerless to help, that was something Sister Carol implicitly understood.

"The love that was there . . . ," Sister Carol thought to herself.

The advice from Jim and the encounter with Robert forced Sister Carol to shift the frame through which she saw her work on the AIDS floors. She no longer focused on the sex, but instead on the tenderness she saw between gay couples. She watched as young men held vigil at their dying lovers' bedsides, never leaving them alone. She saw how effortlessly they vacillated between speaking tenderly when their boyfriends were upset and sarcastically when they needed joy and laughter. Groups of friends visited with regularity, trying desperately to transform the bleak hospital ward into a more genial environment. Love seemed to be everywhere.

"Why is this wrong?" Sister Carol asked herself. She knew what the church taught about gay love. She knew what she was supposed to believe. And yet, she thought, "This can't be wrong. You couldn't say it was wrong."

———

Sister Carol and Sister Mary Ellen spent about six months in New York City. But the way Carol talks about her time at Saint Clare's and Saint Vincent's, working the hotline, meeting people like Will and Jim and Robert, it feels as if it could have been years. When their immersion experience finished, she was not the same person as when she arrived. I asked her about her life up until that point. She hadn't known many gay people in Belleville, and she said she hadn't harbored any resentment toward the gay community. When pressed, she said she had been ignorant, perhaps, and admitted that talking so much about sex made her uncomfortable at first.

Still, I was curious to learn more about what made Carol tick. She has told her stories about New York to friends and family so many times over the years that I think she no longer appreciates that her actions were so radical. A Catholic nun from a small Midwestern city moved to New York to volunteer on AIDS wards at a time when society would rather let young men die in anonymity than offend fragile sensibilities by talking about gay sex. It really was heroic work. But when Carol told me her stories, they sounded too matter-of-fact to me. Was she hiding something? Where was the vulnerability? Why didn't I feel like I was getting the full story? I asked the same question in different ways. I read old newspaper clips to Carol about stigma and bigotry. I hoped to jog her memory, perhaps prompt her to remember how she struggled early on. But she was firm. She did the work because it needed to be done. That was that, it seemed.

But that didn't satisfy me, so I called one of Carol's nephews. When I asked him to describe his Aunt Carol, he pointed out that he never thought of her as a nun, but simply as his aunt. But he said he understood why I might have trouble reading Carol. She was naturally reserved. Quiet, even. But also innately determined and one of the kindest people he'd ever met. He told me a story from when he was younger.

His grandmother, Carol's mom, complained about a young man who lived nearby. He struggled with drug addiction. When he was bored, if he saw Carol's mom out in the yard, he would saunter over for small talk. Carol's mom didn't particularly enjoy these visits and made excuses to cut short the conversations. One Christmas, when Sister Carol gathered together with the rest of the Baltosiewich family at her mom's house, the young man walked over. He struck up a conversation with Sister Carol, who sensed he was a lost soul. Nobody should be alone on Christmas, she thought. So rather than wrapping up the conversation to slip back into the house and enjoy the festivities, Sister Carol invited the young man inside to join the family. She gave him a seat on the couch. Then she sat next to him, listening to his story. Sister Carol's nephew told me his aunt didn't make a big deal of the gesture; she just saw someone in need and did what she could to help. It never really came up again.

Sister Carol met more gay men during those few months in New York than she had ever known in her forty-four years of life. She challenged herself to think not about lifestyles and sex acts and church rules— and instead to focus on love. These were lessons Sister Carol knew she needed if she were to contribute to the fight against HIV back home in Belleville. Seeing the range of services available to people with HIV and AIDS in New York showed Sister Carol the possibilities for ministry back home. She was ready to get started—albeit still frightened of what lay ahead.

11

BORN THIS WAY

Each day when Father Bill McNichols arrived at Saint Vincent's Hospital, he headed to the pastoral care office, where a list awaited him. So many names, so many young people in need of help. Sister Patrice wrote these lists by hand, her impeccable cursive providing Father Bill a call sheet with as many as twenty names a day in those early years of the epidemic. Some of the patients had requested meetings with Father Bill. Others simply needed a checkup. Sometimes Sister Patrice included notes at the bottom of the list. "Mother sits at bedside all afternoon," read one. That image sticks with me. A grieving mother at her dying son's bedside. Maybe she's heartbroken. Maybe she's angry. Maybe she's said something awful to her gay son and now feels guilty. One thing is certain: the situation is heavy, and it's just one of the many emotional encounters awaiting Father Bill.

When I picture Father Bill as a young priest during this time, I imagine him holding these lists. He's talked to me about them many times over the past couple of years, about the heaviness these sheets of paper placed on his soul. Father Bill wasn't content to approach the names as a kind of to-do list, checking off visits as part of some macabre tally. Instead, I picture him contemplating each name, conjuring up details from previous visits. If he didn't recognize a name, he would try to imagine the young man. He knew that most of the men on those lists would likely soon die, but he didn't allow grief to overtake him. At least not yet. During the visits, he asked the patients about their hobbies, what made them laugh. He didn't administer drugs or take vital signs, but he tried his best to make the people on those lists feel human again. People who were in many ways just like him.

———

By the time Father Bill and I speak and text regularly, I know he is openly gay. We talk about his life pretty freely, his calm voice taking me on circuitous journeys through his past, zigging and zagging from his childhood to today and back to the 1980s. From my vantage point, Bill seems comfortable talking about his inner life, including his sexual orientation. He's preached for years that sexual orientation is a core part of identity. He even wrote a letter to the editor arguing that point, published in the *New York Times* in 1984, stating that "homosexuality does indeed matter." So in some ways, Bill's early work in AIDS ministry is unsurprising. Many gay men at the time helped their community. But when Bill sends me a box of old newspaper clippings about his ministry, the personal story of how he came to terms with being a gay priest becomes more complicated.

Inside the box are old photos of Bill as a young Jesuit, before his ordination to the priesthood, his hairstyle and clothes suggesting an embrace of the peace and justice ethos present in some 1970s Catholic circles. Magazine articles from the early 1980s forecast the future for gay Catholics, optimistic that they might be fully accepted in the church. Also tucked inside the box is a newspaper profile of Father Bill's AIDS ministry. This is the reason he's sent me the box; he's mentioned this profile a few times, but I haven't been able to find it on my own.

With the story now in hand, I contact him to set up another interview. On the call, we say hello and catch up for a minute, chatting about the weather, his in New Mexico and mine in Chicago. He tells me about his latest art project, a more-than-life-size crucifix he's labored over for months. He's trying to find it a home.

Then there's a pause. Father Bill jumps in.

"So you want to talk about the 'aversion therapy,' I'm guessing?"

I tend not to disclose specific questions ahead of interviews, preferring instead to let spontaneity drive conversations. But deep inside that article Father Bill has sent me is a section about his coming out experience that he has never mentioned in our hours of previous conversations.

"Sure, if that's OK with you."

Father Bill explains that though he loved being a Jesuit, this early period of his life was not particularly enjoyable. He hasn't talked about this story much over the years, however, and he can't remember why he agreed to open up to a reporter back in the 1980s. The reality, he says, was more complicated than the article suggested.

"But I'll tell you what happened."

————

At school, when Bill was just a child, other students regularly bullied him, the abuse bringing him to tears most days. Bill's classmates called him mean names because he was thin and gentle and, as he put it, he simply "looked gay." In high school, a particular pair of boys was obsessed with picking on him. In front of other students, they ridiculed his mannerisms and laughed at how he carried himself. Afraid that the bullies would corner him on one of the early busses, Bill waited until everyone else was gone and caught the last ride home. When his parents asked where he'd been, he lied and said detention. Then he retreated to his room, where, seeking consolation, he read about the lives of saints, drawing strength from their courage and fostering an early desire to become a priest.

Bill eventually chose to join the Jesuits, which was something of a surprise to those who knew his artistic side. The Jesuits seemed, in a sense, too tough for Bill's personality. But at age nineteen, he headed to the Jesuit novitiate in Florissant, Missouri, to begin his long path to the priesthood.

When he arrived at the house in September 1968, the first Jesuit to greet Bill looked him up and down and stuck out his hand. Bill said hello and reached out. Something changed in the Jesuit's face.

"I'm gonna teach you how to shake hands like a man."

"Oh, God," Bill thought to himself, "more of the same."

Despite the seemingly inauspicious start, Bill loved religious life. He was drawn to the spirituality of Saint Ignatius of Loyola, the founder of the Jesuits, who urged his followers to discover God in all things. One of the older Jesuits wanted the novices to find God in popular culture, so he arranged field trips to movie theaters in nearby St. Louis. *The Lion in Winter. Midnight Cowboy.* And, on one particular evening in 1970 that would prove to be momentous for Bill and some of the other young Jesuit novices, *The Boys in the Band.*

The Boys in the Band revolves around a dinner party hosted by a gay Catholic writer. The cast of characters includes a cadre of gay men, each more or less embodying some kind of gay stereotype: an interior decorator, a couple who can't seem to make monogamy work, a fashion photographer. And then there is Michael, ever the charming host, exploiting the insecurities of his friends for his own entertainment.

Bill stared wide-eyed at the screen. He had known he was different ever since he was a young boy. He once saw an issue of *Life* magazine that included photos of muscly gay men clad in leather. He looked at them, but they didn't do much for him. He told himself that if the men in the magazine embodied homosexuality, and that if he didn't find them particularly attractive, well, he must not be gay. But that night, as he watched Michael and his friends on the big screen, he saw something of himself reflected in the story. Not only that, but he intuited glimpses of the other Jesuits. Bill was experiencing an awakening. Forget about *Life* magazine; Bill realized he was, in fact, gay. It seemed he wasn't the only young Jesuit with that realization, either. On the bus ride home, the normal chatter seemed to retreat as the twenty or so Jesuit novices thought about what they had just seen and what it meant for them.

In the weeks following the movie, Bill wondered if his homosexuality made him unsuited for religious life. He met with one of the older Jesuits, the one who had criticized Bill's handshake, and told him what was going on.

"Well, you need to see a psychologist then, Billy."

Whatever it was that made Bill different seemed throughout his life to have brought him nothing but trouble. He wanted to deal with the issue once and for all, so Bill obeyed the advice of his Jesuit superior.

The Jesuit gave Bill the name of a psychologist who worked with other young men considering religious life. Bill made an appointment. It all seemed easy enough. Bill had no idea that the next several months would be hell.

During their first appointment, the psychologist listened to Bill's story. He then asked if Bill would like to change. There were some exercises, the doctor said, that could repress his attraction to other men. Bill agreed, and the doctor got started.

First, he told Bill to look at photos of naked women in *Playboy* when he masturbated. Bill knew right away this wouldn't work; he couldn't bring himself to sneak copies of the smutty magazine into his Jesuit residence. But he told his superior about the *Playboy* idea. The older Jesuit agreed that it was suboptimal, but he told Bill to continue with the therapy.

At another visit, the psychologist suggested Bill try mind tricks, displaying photos of naked men and then trying to hypnotize him.

"The bile is rising in your chest. You're going to vomit," the therapist repeated over and over.

The psychologist told Bill that the hypnosis would make him nauseous whenever he thought of other men sexually. But that didn't work either. An attractive man still occasionally caught Bill's eye and there was no urge to vomit. Quite the opposite, in fact. But the hypnosis wasn't totally ineffective: it caused him to feel sick before each subsequent therapy session.

With the *Playboy* method a non-starter and the hypnosis failing, the psychologist asked Bill if he wanted to try electricity, a controversial form of "aversion therapy" that, by the early 1970s, had been used to try to "cure" homosexuality for several decades. Bill wasn't sure. When he heard what the process involved—sending volts of electric current through the body with nodes attached to the wrists, ankles, and head—he was spooked. Electricity through his skull? It sounded barbaric.

"What about the ankles and wrists?" the psychologist offered as a compromise.

Bill was reluctant, but he agreed.

The first hour-long session involved one hundred volts passing through his thin body—seventy-five shocks in total. Bill struggled to walk home. When he made it to his room, he put a sock on the door, a sign that no one should bother him under any circumstances. He cried and trembled before finally falling asleep. He didn't leave his room for an entire day.

At the second session, the scene repeated itself. Bill again went home, closed his door, and cried as he tried to forget the horror.

By the time the third session arrived, Bill decided he'd had enough. He walked out.

He tried to convince himself he was "cured," that the two sessions of shock therapy had worked. He was eager to throw himself into religious life, which required a vow of celibacy anyway. What difference did it make if he repressed his sexuality? For eight months, Bill lived as if he were asexual, believing this would enhance his priesthood. But one day, a handsome man walked by and Bill caught himself taking notice—a reaction that sparked in him a mixture of disappointment and fear.

The shock therapy hadn't worked after all.

Bill knew he was traumatized by the "aversion therapy." He told the Jesuit who had arranged the trip to see *The Boys in the Band* about what had happened to him and was taken aback by the priest's anger.

"God made you the way you are," he said.

He told Bill never to see that doctor again.

God made you the way you are. It was one of the first positive affirmations Bill had ever heard about homosexuality. The priest explained that the same energy that aroused sexual attraction also helped foster creativity. He told Bill, who was sharpening his talents as a singer and a painter, that killing his sexuality would simultaneously snuff out his artistry.

"Don't do that."

———

By the time Father Bill started working in AIDS ministry in New York, it felt to him that everyone assumed he was gay. So he just went with it, never denying the gossip about his sexuality. He eventually confirmed the rumors, so that young men with AIDS would know they had an ally. This honesty would eventually harm him. But for now, he saw it as important to his ministry that he be open about his sexual orientation.

His intuition proved to be correct. Sister Patrice Murphy, in her job overseeing the pastoral care department at Saint Vincent's Hospital, said Father Bill was especially gifted in his AIDS chaplaincy precisely because of his own suffering. Among the hundred or so volunteers at the hospital,

Sister Patrice saw Father Bill as unique, because "he knows what it is to suffer, what it is to be young and gay. As a gay male himself, he can empathize, and to some degree make the suffering of those to whom he ministers his own." In Father Bill's suffering, Sister Patrice saw "a model of Christian forgiveness," someone who was able "to survive and be a better person."

———

At Saint Vincent's, Father Bill knew he did not have much time with many of the young men named on those lists. They were once athletic and full of life. Now they lived on an AIDS ward, emaciated after weeks and months of sickness. By the time Father Bill arrived to their rooms, many were too frail to speak. He might pray with them and console their loved ones. But ultimately, the overwhelming majority of the patients died.

The lists weren't particularly memorable, at least not at first glance. Names. Rooms. The date. But each name represented a complex story. These patients were young men, like him, who had moved to New York to pursue their dreams. They left behind hometowns where they didn't feel like they belonged. Bill got to know some of the people named on those lists, including Jeff, a cantor at a university chapel, whose voice touched Father Bill's heart. There was also Louis, who to Bill resembled Saint Aloysius, the young Jesuit who in the sixteenth century had succumbed to plague. Father Bill and Louis talked for hours on the phone each week. Bill recommended spiritual readings, such as those of Saint Thérèse of Lisieux, a suggestion the tough New Yorker initially dismissed. Then one night, Louis called Bill, amazed at the insight of this gentle saint. Father Bill and Louis clicked. But like so many of his friendships in those days, this one came to an end when Bill presided over Louis's funeral Mass.

He knew that many young men who died from AIDS led difficult lives in which they were bullied, made to feel different and less worthy. It was here, in New York, that many of them had finally and fully accepted themselves, relishing the gift of living as openly gay men. And then, just as their lives were falling into place, they were struck down by an illness that brought stigma and condemnation. Father Bill couldn't bring himself to add one more humiliation by throwing their names in the trash. So he didn't. At the end of each day at the hospital, Father Bill held on to his list.

The pile of paper grew larger as the months wore on, the AIDS crisis unrelenting. Tens of thousands of New Yorkers died, many of their names printed on lists now stored in Father Bill's scrapbook. Father Bill soon amassed a hefty pile of dates and names. He thumbed through them, reading some names aloud. When a particularly vivid memory resurfaced, he said a quick prayer. That's when he had an idea.

Father Bill held a special place in his heart for the saints. Stories about their lives had consoled him when he was a child, helping him cope with bullying in school. Now as a young priest, he felt as if the saints were his friends and companions. There's something mystical about Bill's relationship with saints. He doesn't pray *to* them so much as converse *with* them, sharing his fears and hopes. During the height of AIDS, Father Bill sat silently so he could listen for their guidance. They encouraged him to keep going. On the hospital wards, he felt something holy at work. Though society saw the patients as sick men who deserved what they had coming, to Father Bill, they seemed to be saints. He wanted to do something to honor their holy lives.

On the day after All Saints' Day, Catholics observe All Souls' Day, a time set aside to remember loved ones who have died, pray for their salvation, and recall their lives. In times of war or sickness, All Souls' Day could be a source of special comfort to those who had lost loved ones. With the AIDS crisis killing thousands of Americans each year, Father Bill felt like death was everywhere: in the hospitals where he visited patients, in the churches where he celebrated funerals, even in the restaurants and parks where he had passed time with now deceased friends. He needed to do something to remind himself that death would not have the last word, that his friends would be remembered.

Each November 2nd, Father Bill headed to a chapel for All Souls' Day Mass, bringing with him the scrapbook, by now thick with the names of the dead. He placed the book on the altar. As he consecrated the Eucharist, he said a silent prayer for the people named on the lists. He thought of the patients he had befriended before their untimely deaths. He prayed especially for those who died alone, rejected by a society that held their love in such contempt.

12

PRIESTS WITH AIDS

Hundreds of priests gathered on the steps of the Cathedral of Saint
Matthew the Apostle on an April morning in 1987. About twenty-three
years earlier, President John F. Kennedy had lain in repose in the ornate,
marble-walled Washington, DC, church. Today there would be another
funeral Mass.

Soft organ music filled the sanctuary, where more than four hundred
people had gathered to remember Father Michael Peterson. Before Mass,
the priests assembled outside, draped in white robes, waiting for a young
seminarian to lead them down the main aisle. As he walked, he swung a
thurible, releasing incense that soared to the heights of the cathedral. The
organist played and the priests sang loudly—"Oh God, Our Help"—as
they mourned one of their own.

Rumors of Father Mike's declining health had been whispered dis-
creetly through the gay community in Washington before the news made
its way to other priests and then on to the popular press. In those days,
a call from an archbishop could delay a story from going to print, which

is why Father Mike's death had been a shock to so many Catholics: they had no idea that he had lived a double life.

Father Mike had been a talented medical doctor, specializing in psychiatry. He entered seminary later than most, already in his thirties. He taught college for a while. But he wanted to use his medical background to help priests and nuns struggling with addiction and mental health. So he founded a hospital to treat addiction, and later, priests who sexually abused minors. There was never a shortage of clients. Through that work, Father Mike had befriended bishops and priests from throughout the United States. He traveled frequently, though he seemed to demur when asked to speak at events hosted by gay and lesbian Catholics. And now, at just forty-four, Father Mike was being laid to rest.

Archbishop James Hickey presided over the funeral Mass. He had grown close to Father Mike, visiting him in the hospital nearly every day as his body grew weak. Like many bishops in the 1980s, Hickey toed the line when it came to homosexuality, cracking down on dissent in his archdiocese. But he also had a pastoral side. When Father Mike got sick, the archbishop reached out and the priest told him the truth: he was dying from AIDS.

The archbishop, though soft-spoken and reserved himself, urged Father Mike to go public about the true nature of his illness. He didn't want one of his priests to live in secrecy and shame. It took some cajoling, but Father Mike agreed, and he wrote a letter to every bishop in the country, making them aware of his diagnosis and letting them know his time was nearing its end.

At Father Mike's funeral, Archbishop Hickey spoke openly about his illness.

"His last gift to us," the archbishop said, "was a stark reminder of the human dimensions of this terrible epidemic, that those who suffer from it are our brothers and sisters who deserve our care, respect, and support."

The archbishop compared those reeling from AIDS to Christ's own passion and death.

It was 1987, a gay Catholic priest had died from AIDS, and his archbishop compared him to Christ. The moment wasn't lost on the young seminarian swinging the incense. Tears filled his eyes.

At the end of Mass, a bronze casket with Father Mike's remains was escorted down the long aisle, the organ loud enough to muffle the crying of his friends and colleagues. As the congregation exited, a reporter interviewed another priest on the steps of the cathedral, asking how he wanted to remember his friend. He spoke kindly of Father Mike.

"If this had to happen to anyone, Michael was the one to teach the church a lot through his illness," he said.

But when the reporter asked for his name, the priest demurred. Nationally, Americans were growing a bit more comfortable talking about HIV. Rock Hudson had died from AIDS in 1985, the same year that President Reagan had finally broken his silence about the disease while responding to a reporter's question. The AIDS quilt was being assembled in San Francisco. But on the steps of that cathedral, a priest refused to give his name to a reporter. Father Mike may have gone public about his illness, but when it came to AIDS in the celibate Catholic priesthood, silence prevailed.

———

Learning about AIDS affecting priests and brothers elicited within me a range of emotions. News stories from the time tend to adopt one of two tones. Often, articles focused on the compassion from bishops shown to priests who were dying from AIDS, such as Archbishop Hickey's pastoral response to Father Mike Peterson. That seemed to be the norm, at least in private. Publicly, that understanding only went so far.

Even Archbishop Hickey, who had tried to silence a gay Catholic organization in 1984 but who later compared Peterson's suffering to Jesus's, told a reporter a few days after the priest's death that even as "the AIDS epidemic grows, we have to remain firm in our Catholic teaching." Other stories skewed entirely more salacious. After all, priests take a vow of celibacy, and the church is conservative when it comes to sexual morality. So stories about AIDS affecting the priesthood, with the seemingly inherent hypocrisy, were easily sensationalized. A priest engaging in an affair with a woman can create many challenges, including the shame that results from failing to live up to his vows and the emotional toll the affair may place on his partner. But for a gay priest who contracted HIV through sex with another man, the shame and stigma are heightened because of the church's teaching against homosexuality.

Gay Catholics at the time seemed torn about what to make of the phenomenon. Early on, bishops and priests tried to hide the true nature of how a priest died when the real reason was AIDS, even using their influence to alter death certificates with a cause of death that they felt was less controversial, such as pneumonia or cancer. Some of these same church leaders regularly condemned homosexuality, even while privately showing sympathy to their many gay priests. I could sense that concern when reading the stories decades later. When it turned out that this same storyline played out in a place that is important to me today, it caused me to look more closely at the complexity the topic embodies, even into the present day.

———

While researching this project, the history of AIDS and the Catholic Church became enmeshed with my daily life. What I read, the people I met, and the experiences I underwent changed the way I thought about what it means today to be gay and Catholic, long before I finally sat down to write these pages. As I learned more of this history—my own community's history—I reflected on my faith life. Learning about communities of LGBT Catholics in the 1980s made me realize that I missed being a part of a parish. I attended Mass regularly, but I snuck in as the opening hymn ended, kept to myself, and then left before meeting any other parishioners.

A couple of years into researching this book, my partner and I hopped around to different Chicago parishes each Sunday morning, eager to explore new neighborhoods and perhaps find a faith community that felt authentically welcoming. On a whim, we visited an oddly shaped church in a nearby neighborhood, the building constructed with street-level, clear-glass windows, so walkers are able to look inside and see the sanctuary. The congregation itself is small enough that the greeters this particular Sunday noticed we were new. One of them asked us to bring up the bread and wine for the priest to consecrate before communion. It was a welcoming gesture, albeit not one I particularly loved. I still preferred the anonymity granted by soaring, more traditional churches. This place, evidently, was not that. Still, that the greeter asked a gay couple visiting the parish for the first time to be part of the Mass felt encouraging.

When the time came to make the short walk from the back of the church up the center aisle to the altar, the priest greeted us. He took the bread and wine and offered us a blessing. Another good sign.

We cut short our "church shopping" and returned to this parish. The music was lively and soulful, the homilies passionate and challenging. With some prodding from my partner, I even came to appreciate the small feel, eventually recognizing regulars each week and being noticed in return. I observed that among the various ministries active at the parish, which seemed to be heavily clustered around food—a soup kitchen, a food pantry, meal delivery—there was no group explicitly geared toward LGBT Catholics. Though it was a modestly sized community, there were a number of young gays and lesbians, including a few other couples, who attended each week. The parish was clearly welcoming, but I wondered why a community so focused on social justice seemed to lack what is now a pretty common—at least in some places—parish ministry.

But as we approached Valentine's Day, I began to understand. The pastor, an energetic white priest in his sixties who had sharpened his preaching skills while serving a Black Catholic parish on Chicago's south side, spoke at the end of Mass. The announcements sometimes took on a life of their own. They also provided the pastor a chance to give something of a second homily, delivering remarks he might have forgotten while he was preaching.

"Around Valentine's Day, the church has a tradition of blessing married couples," he said. "So we'll do that next week. It's easy; couples will stand up and I'll bless you."

Nothing out of the ordinary. I had seen this ritual play out at other parishes. It's kind of hokey, though perhaps meaningful to married couples. But then the priest added a few words, quickly, trying to wrap up.

"Anyone is welcome to stand up for the blessing," he said. "Gay, straight, divorced-and-remarried. It doesn't matter."

That was it. The priest offered a final blessing, and the recessional hymn began. We were done. But those words bounced around in my head. They didn't seem particularly challenging for the pastor. He didn't stammer or read from notes. Nothing suggested that this invitation was out of the ordinary. But in my more than thirty years of going to Mass, I had never heard anything like those words.

In my experience, priests had only talked about gay marriage in order to denounce it, often on the internet, or to privately tell me they supported it but could never preach that in public. Yet here was a priest who, with just a few words, smashed to bits the idea that gay couples were somehow second class in the church. And he did so without ever explicitly challenging church teaching or even singling out gay Catholics. We were simply part of the parish, invited to participate in the silly

Valentine's Day blessing like anyone else. Put another way, the parish was fully welcoming and, when it came to sexuality, it seemed to be fully integrated. We knew we had found our parish home, a place that suggested maybe it was indeed possible to make these two identities work.

Several months later, now deep into my research, I discovered by chance that the inclusive nature of our new parish home was no accident. It was created intentionally, a few decades ago by a forward-thinking priest who wanted a space where all people felt welcome. That priest, parishioners later found out, was himself gay. And like many gay men in the 1980s, he was vulnerable to the growing epidemic.

———

Father Jim Noone had wanted to be a priest for as long as he could remember. The best way he could describe his calling as a high school seminarian was to say that he was simply attracted to the idea of helping other people. That's what priests did, so that's what he wanted to be. On Thursdays, when seminarians were given a day off, Jim and a group of friends went to the Cabrini-Green housing project in Chicago. The series of buildings—named for Mother Frances Cabrini, the first US citizen to be canonized by the Catholic Church—that opened to great fanfare in the middle of the twentieth century was by the 1970s in great disrepair. Violence was common, and the exteriors were crumbling. For the kids who lived in the complex, gangs were always a threat. Jim wanted to assist the residents who strived to keep their community strong in spite of the challenges, so he and his friends volunteered at an after-school program. Each week, they taught religious education. It didn't matter that most of the children weren't Catholic; the point of the program was to give them a safe place to go after school.

When he graduated from high school seminary, Jim enrolled at Mundelein Seminary. Far from Cabrini-Green, located in the northern Chicago suburbs, the seminary's architecture reinforces the notion that the young seminarians are on retreat from a chaotic and hurting world. Large red-brick buildings dot a well-manicured lawn and small pedestrian bridges cut across ponds and through gardens that color the grounds. There's even a golf course, so future priests can learn to be gentlemen, grow-ing comfortable socializing with the doctors and lawyers and investors who comprise Chicago's professional class. But Jim wanted more than that.

After ordination, he sought creative ways to help people in need. At one point, he considered the church's teaching against abortion. He thought to himself, "If we consider it a sin, what are we doing to help pregnant women in need?" Not enough, he realized. To help fix that, he volunteered with a program that provided money and support to young women in need. When he saw children with special needs were left out of religious education, he supported a program that would be inclusive and welcoming, reminding the youngsters that they were "God's special friends." His sense of humor and dedication to parish ministry won him respect from fellow priests, who elected him to lead the Association of Chicago Priests in 1984.

The following year, on a warm summer evening, Jim and a friend were watching television. A newscaster talked about the increasing number of AIDS diagnoses in Chicago, which at that point stood at about 250. The numbers were far lower than in other cities such as New York and San Francisco, but they were a sign of things to come. Two-hundred and fifty lives forever changed.

"I'll bet 125 of those are Catholic," Jim guessed. He asked his friend if the church was doing anything in response.

"Why don't you do something?"

It was a good question. Why didn't Father Jim do something?

Over the next few months, he sought out information about HIV and AIDS to see how parishes and priests might be of help. He learned that while individual Catholics were already undertaking heroic work, they seemed to be laboring alone, not part of a broader network that could share resources and provide moral support. Soon after, Saint Joseph's, a Catholic hospital located near Boystown, hosted a conference about HIV and AIDS. Jim attended, listening to activists talk about the challenges facing people with AIDS. He stuck around and asked questions.

A group of young faith leaders who also participated in the hospital seminar met again a few weeks later. By working together, they reasoned, they could accomplish more. The need was great already and was expected to grow. They decided to organize the AIDS Pastoral Care Network. Jim joined the board, intent on learning all he could about HIV and AIDS, while worrying in secret how the disease was affecting a community well-known to him.

The next year, 1986, Jim was assigned to be a pastor at a small church not too far from both the housing project where he had volunteered as a young seminarian and the Boystown bars he now sometimes visited on his days off. The parish was diverse, with a mixture of Irish, German, and Puerto Rican Catholics. They all worshipped together at Jim's new parish, situated along a stretch of Armitage Avenue that was home to a number of small restaurants and coffee shops—places that people bragged about, describing them to their friends as "a great little hole in the wall." Regulars talked about these establishments with a sense of ownership, as if they had discovered some previously unknown gem. Jim picked up on that sense of pride in the neighborhood as he set out to make the parish "a great little hole-in-the-wall church." The idea was simple. Nearby parishes, massive and wealthier, seemed to get all the attention, but Father Jim's new church was small and nimble. It could transform and meet the needs of a changing community.

———

Though the Chicago archbishop's relationship to the local gay community had been strained, Cardinal Joseph Bernardin nonetheless released a statement calling on parishes to "open their doors and their hearts to those touched in any way by AIDS, as well as to their friends and family." Given the proximity of his parish to Boystown, Father Jim and a group of like-minded pastors made a special effort to reach out to Chicago's gay and lesbian community, just as HIV and AIDS moved in.

One of the first outreach activities resembled a project Father Bill McNichols was undertaking in New York around the same time. In October 1987, Father Jim's church hosted a healing Mass for people with AIDS. Tension lingered between the gay community and the Catholic hierarchy. It had only been a year since the Vatican reiterated its hardline stance condemning homosexuality. In Chicago, Cardinal Bernardin had attempted a more moderate approach to gay and lesbian issues, keeping in regular contact with leaders in the gay Catholic community, but he had also opposed gay civil rights laws, enraging many gay activists who believed the church's political clout had stymied progress. Father Jim understood the anger. The whole situation frustrated him, too, because what he saw in parishes was so different than the clashes he read about in the news.

"The hierarchical statements basically have very little to do with day-to-day things in the parish," he told the *Windy City Times*, a gay newspaper. "When people are in need, people in the parish want to do what they can to respond."

Through his ministry, Father Jim had seen Catholics step up when people became sick. Parishioners cooked and cleaned for people who needed help at home and provided rides to medical appointments. Some brought Communion to the homebound and others simply visited, attempting to combat the loneliness that so often accompanies illness. Father Jim thought that this type of ministry would transfer easily into a new ministry for people with AIDS, but he also understood that he would have to convince the wider gay community that they could trust Catholics.

"I don't think we have a handle yet on how to deal with the alienation," he said of gay people hurt by the church's views on homosexuality. "Sometimes it seems like every time we take a step forward, a statement [from the hierarchy] comes out and we step back."

Father Jim decided gay Catholics should know they weren't alone in their struggles. Allies in parishes felt as angry about the church's statements on homosexuality as they did. And they wanted to offer a welcoming space to their LGBT friends and family. To help get that message across, Father Jim advertised his church in gay newspapers. He mentioned gay and lesbian people in his homilies, so visitors would know they were welcome. And he prayed for people with AIDS regularly, a small gesture to call attention to the growing crisis.

As for the AIDS healing Mass, Father Jim wanted to make sure the entire community was aware of the opportunity to gather together for prayer. Through his work with the AIDS Pastoral Care Network, Father Jim knew HIV and AIDS were a growing issue among gay Hispanics, some of whom worshipped at his church. This rising crisis too often went unnoticed by white gay activists, he realized. As he had pointed out in a report he helped draft for the cardinal in 1986, one in ten people in Chicago diagnosed with AIDS was Hispanic, and there were often few resources available for Catholic Spanish-speaking communities, where homophobia could be crushing. So Father Jim decided that part of the healing service would be in Spanish. He had high hopes for the Mass.

The service, he said, could be "a real opportunity for the Catholic Church to meet the gay community." That, Father Jim thought, "could be healing for both. I imagine our parish is going to be transformed by this experience."

Father Jim was also undergoing a transformation of his own.

His illness was becoming more difficult to hide. Where he once had a full face and joked with friends about struggling to keep a handle on his weight, he was becoming thin. A parish secretary noticed how frail he looked, and she hadn't remembered him previously taking so many pills. That was when Father Jim knew he had to begin telling his friends the truth.

While spending time with a priest with whom he had been close friends since their seminary work at Cabrini-Green, Father Jim said he had something important to say.

"I'm sick," he said. "I tested positive for HIV."

"Oh God, Jim," his friend replied. "You have AIDS?"

"No, AIDS is when the HIV sort of takes hold," Jim told his friend, trying to help him overcome his shock by explaining the medical reality in a way that might make sense. "That's when all the symptoms and illnesses arise. Right now, I'm just HIV-positive."

Jim asked if his friend wanted to know how he contracted HIV; the friend shook his head no. But he had other questions. He thought Jim had actually been looking healthier than he had in a while, going to the gym more regularly and losing weight. He asked Jim about this.

Jim explained that since there was no reliable medicine to help with HIV, his doctors had suggested he stay healthy by exercising and eating well. Anything he could do to support his immune system might be beneficial in slowing the progression from HIV to AIDS. It seemed to work for a while. People had commented that he looked good. But now, Jim could tell his body was beginning to fail him. He felt tired and he was growing weak. He had watched others die from AIDS, and he knew how their immune systems betrayed them, leaving them vulnerable to common illnesses. Pneumonia that an otherwise healthy young man should be able to fight off was suddenly lethal. Young men who once visited the gym four or five times a week were now consigned to bed, reliant on others for simple tasks like eating and bathing. Jim wanted his friend to know he was sick in case it came to that.

Jim also confided to his friend another secret. He was gay. His friend suddenly recalled a certain night when Jim showed him photos from a trip to the Grand Canyon.

One picture had stood out. Jim, wearing jeans and a plaid shirt along with a cowboy hat and boots, stood next to another man who also dressed the part. Jim and the other man in the photo may have been going for a butch cowboy look, but his friend thought he had seen for a quick second something else in that picture that he hadn't articulated that night.

Now, with Jim revealing that he was gay and that he had HIV, it all clicked. Jim's trip to the Grand Canyon must have been a vacation with his boyfriend. The man in the photo, he later learned, had previously died from AIDS. Jim had been with him, right until the very end.

Father Jim Noone's story began circulating among Chicago priests, including some of Jim's friends. Some had already known about Jim's double life and they offered to be supportive in his time of need. Many others, however, now seemed scared to be around him. They were embarrassed to be associated with him and reluctant even to acknowledge the truth. Shame seemed to be everywhere.

Though Jim felt tired and weak as the virus took its toll, he wanted to continue his ministry. Being with his flock meant too much to him. He saw their pain and wanted to help. His own could wait.

———

That priests were not immune to HIV and AIDS was fairly well known by the late 1980s. By the time Father Mike Peterson's funeral was held in April 1987, news reports of other priests battling HIV and AIDS had already been published across the country, including in newspapers in Boston, Chicago, San Francisco, and New York.

One of the first accounts was printed in 1985. A priest of the Diocese of Worcester, Massachusetts, had died from AIDS in October, at just forty-one. His family thought he died from a brief bout with cancer. But the real cause of death was leaked by hospital staff who saw it printed on his death certificate. Reporters in Boston picked up on the story, which eventually spread by wire services into newspapers all over the United States. Devoutly Catholic, his family was shocked to hear a radio news report revealing his true cause of death.

A January 1987 story in the *National Catholic Reporter* recounted the death of a Franciscan priest who left his New York friary in 1980, moved to San Francisco to live as an openly gay man, and later contracted HIV. When he developed AIDS, his Franciscan community flew him back to New York and cared for him until his death.

The *Los Angeles Times* addressed the taboo topic of gays in the priesthood the following month, with a number of former priests and sociologists pointing out that it appeared likely the percentage of priests who were homosexual was significantly higher than the general population. The exact number of priests who identified as gay, and among those, who were sexually active, was impossible to pinpoint. But that same year, the *National Catholic Reporter* published a series of stories about homosexuality in the priesthood, in which a researcher suggested that as many as 26 percent of priests were gay, while some seminarians and priests guessed that a majority of seminarians were gay. The implication was that even if just a small percentage of gay priests broke their vows, HIV and AIDS could present an ongoing challenge for the priesthood.

By this point, HIV was already an epidemic in gay communities in New York and San Francisco. The number of cases was rising fast in so-called second-wave cities such as Chicago. Church leaders throughout the United States were urged to take the disease more seriously by educating clergy about ways to protect themselves.

In some places, it appeared education for sexually active priests would come too late. An article in the *Village Voice* reported that at least four priests in New York City had died from AIDS, though a spokesman for the archdiocese denied it. Claiming ignorance about the existence of gay priests, let alone priests with AIDS, was a common tactic for church leaders in the 1980s. A spokesman for the National Conference of Catholic Bishops called the claim that priests tended to be gay at higher rates than the general population "baloney."

While some bishops stood by their priests after a diagnosis of HIV, supporting them publicly and visiting them at home or in the hospital, others meted out severe punishments. In Atlanta, priests who were diagnosed with AIDS had their fitness for the priesthood questioned, as church leaders pondered whether a priest with HIV could sufficiently condemn homosexuality. In Houston, a doctor said he had treated three Catholic priests for HIV and that he was stunned when they each were thrown out of their rectories because of their illness.

Still, though rarely, some church leaders did push bishops to acknowledge the reality that many priests were gay, including some who were sexually active and thus at risk for HIV infection.

"There's no use putting our heads in the sand," Bishop Emerson J. Moore, an auxiliary bishop in New York, said in February 1987. "This is a problem that's affecting us, and we just have to be ready for it." Bishop Moore's insight came from firsthand experience, as he shared a rectory with a priest who had recently been diagnosed with HIV.

In many ways, Bishop Moore's admonition that the church take AIDS seriously was an extension of his zeal for social justice. He had spoken out publicly against racial injustice for decades. As a young Black priest in 1967, he condemned the church as a racist institution. Later, he was arrested while protesting against apartheid. His ministry attracted attention, and Pope John Paul II visited his Harlem church in 1979. He was made a bishop in 1982, and in 1990, he signed a letter calling for change in the church, including the introduction of women priests and further developing the church's teaching on human sexuality.

Bishop Moore also struggled for years with drug addiction, something he spoke openly about to others he met in rehab. When he died in 1995, at just fifty-seven, the Archdiocese of New York said in a statement that he had succumbed to "natural causes of unknown origin." That puzzled those who had long suspected that Moore had been living with HIV. When questioned, the archdiocese did not deny that the bishop had died from AIDS. But church leaders did not admit it either, saying they could only repeat the information provided on Moore's death certificate, which stated that the deceased bishop was a "laborer" who died from "unknown natural causes." Later, an AIDS activist petitioned to have Moore's death certificate updated to indicate that he had died from AIDS-related complications.

It's impossible to know how many bishops read the various newspaper stories circulating in January and February 1987 about priests with AIDS. But they were made aware through other channels that HIV presented a challenge to their priests by March of that year, when Father Mike Peterson's letter arrived.

"I hope that in my own struggle with this disease, in finally acknowledging that I have this lethal syndrome, there might come some measure of compassion, understanding, and healing for me and for others with it—especially those who face this disease alone and in fear."

―――

By 1989, when Father Jim Noone revealed he was HIV-positive to his priest friends, leaders in the Archdiocese of Chicago had been made aware that HIV and AIDS were affecting its priests, even if they weren't quite ready to acknowledge that reality publicly. An internal archdiocesan memo marked "RESTRICTED USE" was published on December 1, 1990, World AIDS Day. Titled "Archdiocesan Resources for Priests with AIDS," the memo laid out how the archdiocese would respond if a priest disclosed his HIV status.

Much of the memo was affirming: it said priests who were HIV-positive or sick with AIDS must receive "understanding and unconditional, non-judgmental support." The memo acknowledged that the stigma that often accompanied HIV could "create a sense of failure and spiritual bankruptcy" in priests affected by the virus and pledged to counter that with support teams. Church leaders in Chicago promised to allow priests to continue carrying out their ministry so long as they felt well, and to support them financially and continue to provide health insurance. They also promised, when possible, to help non-clergy "who, through contact with a priest, has also become HIV infected."

The memo also reiterated church teaching on celibacy. Even if authorities were willing to care for priests who became sick through a sexual encounter, chastity was still the rule. The memo stated that the church "must reaffirm efforts to create structures that will support a truly human and celibate life in service of the Church."

Though the policy seemed to signal good intentions, it hinted at the trepidation church leaders felt about publicly disclosing that priests were affected by HIV and AIDS, especially because they were supposed to remain celibate. The document was created "to prevent hasty and hurtful decisions impacting both the Archdiocese and the individual HIV-infected priests." Those who wished to go public about their HIV status were instructed to "first discuss this with the Vicar for Priests" as such an announcement "would involve not only himself but the diocese as well." Together, they would "discern the appropriateness and manner of disclosure."

As the days grew shorter and the cold settled on Chicago in 1990, Father Jim Noone felt weak. It was November, with the busy Advent season just around the corner. By this point, many in the parish knew he was HIV-positive and understood he might not be alive to celebrate Christmas with the community. But Father Jim's private goal was to persevere so that he could revel in the community he had helped build one last time.

Though by this point quite sick, Father Jim received permission from the cardinal to remain in ministry at the parish and to live in his room at the rectory until the end. Getting through the four weeks of Advent was a challenge, but Christmas Day had finally arrived. Father Jim summoned the energy to celebrate Mass with his parishioners, sitting on a stool placed behind the altar when he became fatigued.

After Mass, Father Jim's brother picked him up for Christmas dinner. Jim was a devoted uncle who loved visiting his extended family. Aware that this might be his last Christmas with them, he put his pain aside and climbed into the car. But his brother was saddened by the physical pain Jim displayed.

"You know, Jim, I always thought you had lived such a charmed life," his brother said, now more aware of the physical and emotional struggles Jim had faced and of the challenges that remained. Despite his pain, Jim was still quick and charming. Without missing a beat, he replied, "I still am."

By late January, Father Jim's health had deteriorated significantly. Friends and family gathered at the rectory on an icy January night. Jim drifted in and out of consciousness. Some of Jim's family left to get coffee, leaving him alone in the rectory with his brother. Father Jim smiled when his brother took his hand and told him it was OK to let go, that the fight was over.

———

One of Father Jim's colleagues held vigil in his friend's church, just steps from the room where the young priest lay dying. He had revered Jim, who had supported and mentored him as a young priest. When Jim had breathed his last, at just forty-three, sadness enveloped him, but he later found comfort in his realization that Father Jim's heavy burdens were through, that the shame and guilt and fear he knew his friend suffered would not follow him into the next life.

Father Jim had eventually become "unafraid of the truth," as another friend put it, and toward the end of his life, he insisted on total transparency.

Father Jim didn't want AIDS to be the focus of his funeral sermon, but before he died, he asked his friend who would preach about his life to state the true cause of his death, a gesture to show others who suffered silently with HIV and AIDS that they should not feel any shame. Church leaders urged the homilist to reconsider, but he refused. Father Jim's friends and family were awed by his act of courage.

The final request was in keeping with Father Jim's approach to the disease and to his faith.

"There is a tendency to give up hope when facing AIDS," he said in 1987, a few years before his death. "But Christ's presence says, 'Don't give up hope.' There is a tendency to fear. Christ's presence says, 'We are not alone.' There is a tendency to wonder, 'Why is God doing this to me, to us?' Christ's presence says, 'God hates this virus as much as we do.'"

13

FRIENDS OF DOROTHY

Everything had been planned just perfectly. The three-bedroom house, overlooking matured oak and evergreen trees on the horizon, had been fully renovated. Inside the white framed house with its red-tile roof was a new kitchen. A second bathroom had been added, and out back, a new deck overlooked the hills, a creek, and the colorful flowerbeds. Taken together, the home was ready to welcome those seeking refuge from a weary world.

But there was one problem: nobody wanted to move in.

Nestled alongside a quiet golf course in Oakland, California, the house had been specially retrofitted as a place where terminally ill people could spend their final weeks and months. Specifically, Catholic priests with AIDS.

The idea was straightforward enough. Church leaders in Oakland had heard horror stories about priests with AIDS who were afraid to go public with their illness. In some instances, they had no place to live once their religious superiors learned they were sick. In response, the Diocese of Oakland partnered with three male religious orders and the Sisters of Mercy to fund the house, convinced they could interest sick priests from the West Coast to fill the three bedrooms immediately. From there, they would be able to offer the rooms to other priests on a rolling basis. The house opened, so to speak, in January 1990. A few days later, the former Catholic brother in charge of managing the house had received few inquiries. News about the house seemed to be getting around, but the priests who called were frightened, battered down by shame and stigma.

"They'd only give us their first name," he recalled. "They would say that no one knows except their doctors. Some were afraid they would lose their health benefits, some were afraid they'd lose their pensions. It is part of the fear of coming forward. No one wants to talk about it."

Unable to place any West Coast priests in the house, the search went national, with letters to bishops and religious superiors delivered throughout the country. An openly gay priest who had tried to collect stories about other priests with AIDS was consulted, but he had no names. There was "a conspiracy of silence" around the issue, he said, invoking the slain gay civil rights hero Harvey Milk. Priests with AIDS suffered from stigma and mistreatment, and they just weren't willing to share their stories, even with other priests who promised discretion.

The search continued for a few more months. In the meantime, the house remained empty. The nearly $80,000 that the diocese and religious orders had sunk into renovations, making it more livable with handicap-accessible amenities, seemed to be a waste. That didn't sit well with Michael Harank, a nurse and a gay Catholic who had arrived in California a few years earlier, moving from Boston where he had worked on a hospital AIDS ward. He had accepted a job with an AIDS nonprofit in Oakland serving primarily African American men. He was the only white member of the staff. He visited patients in their homes and did what he could to help make them comfortable.

Because of his background in AIDS medicine and his connection to a Catholic social justice movement, it didn't take long for local church leaders to ask Michael if he would lend a hand in trying to identify priests with AIDS. He signed on as a medical advisor, happy to assist even if he thought the prospects for finding residents were dim.

"I think this is a wonderful and merciful and beautiful idea," he told the group backing the house. "But I don't think you're going to get a response."

After all, Michael knew intimately how complicated the issue of homosexuality was in the Catholic Church.

———

Michael had graduated in 1976 with a degree in religion from the Jesuit-run College of the Holy Cross in Massachusetts, where he first joined the Catholic Worker. Dorothy Day and Peter Maurin founded the organization in the 1930s, publishing a newspaper for laborers and the unemployed to spread word of the church's solidarity with the poor during the Great Depression. In the decades that followed, the Catholic Worker led a pacifist movement and founded "houses of hospitality" that provided meals and shelters to those without means, foregoing available government funding as a way of staying true to its anti-war stance and relying instead on freewill donations to sustain its work.

In the late 1970s, Michael spent time with the aging Dorothy Day, a woman many considered even then to be a saint. He helped her answer correspondence and learned firsthand what it meant to be a social gospel–oriented Catholic. That experience also gave him insight into the limits of how welcoming even the most hospitable of Catholic bastions could be when it came to homosexuality.

Michael was an editor for the organization's newspaper, the *Catholic Worker*. In 1971, the paper had published an editorial condemning anti-Semitism. Columns like that were common in the *Worker*, part of its mission to call attention to societal injustices. But the piece prompted a response from a young gay man who wanted to know why the *Worker* hadn't stood up for gay people, who were regularly experiencing discrimination, especially as a result of the growing backlash against the push for gay rights.

"If the *Catholic Worker* is the gentle enemy of all oppressors of people, the pages of this newspaper have been silent on the increased oppression, discrimination, and violence taking place against American gay people," he wrote. The letter writer added that he was puzzled and saddened by the oversight.

A debate broke out among the group of young editors, including Michael, about whether to publish the letter. Though Day had previously lived a Bohemian lifestyle, one that embraced sexual liberation, she took seriously her conversion to Catholicism. She was a daughter of the church, which inspired both her radical commitment to the poor as well as her orthodoxy around traditional sexual morality, which included her views on homosexuality. In her private diary, in 1975, she wrote that her "heart [was] troubled" by the mere mention of homosexuality, or "unnatural sex," as she put it. She cited the advice of Saint Paul, writing, "Let these things be not so much as mentioned amongst you."

It's not that Day didn't know and even care for gay people, many of whom were active in the Catholic Worker movement. She sometimes stood up for them, albeit quietly, like the time she admonished a volunteer, reminding him that "*Someone* has to minister to gay people." She seemed torn, noting that the issue of gay relationships had been "judged with horror and coldness" by some Catholic Workers but also recognizing the "faithful friendship which endured till death" among some gays and lesbians. But she demanded discretion, especially for volunteers in same-sex relationships. (Another gay volunteer had been asked to leave his Catholic Worker community after spending too much time on the phone with a boyfriend; his transgression seemed not that he was gay, but what Day apparently interpreted as his tactlessness.)

Publishing a letter that seemed to call out the church, however gently, for its negative views on homosexuality would violate Day's prohibition on covering this topic, along with birth control and abortion, in her newspaper. So an editor took the letter to Day, who by this point was nearing the end of her life and had little to do with the day-to-day operations of the newspaper she had founded. But out of a sense of respect for her legacy, the editor, a gay man himself, visited her at her cottage on Staten Island. He wanted to know if she supported the publication of the letter.

Day's ambivalent response took him by surprise. Like she had previously in her diary, she quoted Saint Paul, invoking not the passages often used to condemn homosexuality, but his words urging people to refrain from discussing it. She pointed out that the newspaper had hardly addressed every social ill in the United States, as the young reader had suggested in his letter. But she also told the editor that the *Worker* was now his and his team's and that they could do whatever they wanted with the letter.

The editor decided not to publish it. If Dorothy Day had demanded discretion on the issue of homosexuality during her long tenure heading the movement, they would honor her wishes in this instance as well.

———

That experience had unsettled Michael, who as a gay man possessed a viewpoint that was simply alien to Day and other heterosexual Catholics. A few years later, he left his Catholic Worker community in New York for another in Boston, which he knew to be more welcoming to gay and lesbian volunteers. More than a decade after the letter incident, as he visited people with AIDS in Oakland, Michael recalled how that kind of institutionalized and implicit homophobia infected even the most well-meaning of Catholics. There was no way, he thought, that priests would be willing to come out as gay, tell the world they had HIV and AIDS, and

then pack up and move into a new home—no matter how nicely mani-
cured the gardens or discreet the location. It just wasn't going to happen.
But, he wondered, why should the house sit empty?

Through his AIDS work in Oakland's African American communities, Michael was well aware of the need for residential hospices in the
city, and there weren't nearly enough rooms in Oakland, where in addition to AIDS, the crack cocaine crisis was hitting the city's poor with a
fury. He spoke to his colleagues who were trying to find priests to move
into the empty house and put forward an idea: a Catholic Worker house
for people with AIDS.

Across the country, HIV had wreaked havoc on communities of color,
a reality dating back to the earliest years of the epidemic. In 1985, African Americans accounted for 25 percent of new AIDS diagnoses, even
though they comprised just about 12 percent of the total population. In
1990, the number of new HIV infections among African Americans was
higher than it was among whites, and by 1994, the death rate from HIV
infection for young Black men was four times as high as white men.
In Alameda County, where Oakland sits, more than 50 percent of new
AIDS diagnoses were among people of color and the city didn't have a
single residential hospice to serve people with AIDS. In his proposal,
Michael wrote, "this picture of terrible poverty and oppression leaves me
with an overwhelming sense of sadness and anger." He sought to channel
his emotions into action.

"I could fill this house in a week," Michael told his colleagues matter-
of-factly, "with people who are homeless and without families."

He created a plan that drew from his previous experiences. He had
lived at two other Catholic Worker houses, in Boston and New York. He
had cared for terminally ill patients for more than a decade, first people
dying from cancer and now from AIDS. He had witnessed the suffering
that accompanied dying alone in a hospital room, or worse, abandoned to
the streets. He wanted to use the empty residence to serve homeless and

low-income people with AIDS. He'd live nearby and give each resident a private room. All he asked from the church was free use of the house. The original goal of the backers had been to serve people with AIDS, he reminded them. Since priests seemed uninterested in moving, why not open it up to others in need?

"There was no shortage of people who were abandoned by their families, had no place to go, and were dying in hospitals alone," he recalled.

Within two weeks, Michael identified three people who would be good candidates for the house and asked them if they would like to move in.

That summer, the first guest arrived to the Bethany House of Hospitality, whose mission was "to create a sanctuary of peace and compassionate care." A Vietnam War veteran from San Francisco, Henry had a long history of drug abuse and was into a hard-core sex scene. Now he was sick, diagnosed with HIV, and he had nowhere to live. He was astonished when he was given his own room in a nicely appointed home overlooking the California hills. He stayed for more than three years, during which time he and Michael became friends, even marching together in anti-war protests. Other guests spent just a few months, including Damon, a twenty-nine-year-old African American man who was deaf and thought to be mute.

Damon had fled a squalid single-room-occupancy hotel before moving into the house. Once he felt safe in his new home, he began speaking, no longer afraid that others would ridicule his voice. Michael scrounged up the resources to help Damon fulfill his final wish: a day trip with his dad to ride the Giant Dipper roller coaster on the Santa Cruz Beach Boardwalk. When Damon died, a man who once counted not a single friend was celebrated by more than fifty people at a funeral service held in the house's backyard.

Michael had seen how some other Catholic homes for people with AIDS fell short. He had visited Mother Teresa's hospice across the bay in San Francisco. Though the order provided beds for people with AIDS who lacked financial resources, like her order's other residences in New York and Washington, DC, the San Francisco residence could be excruciatingly uncomfortable, with a focus on simplicity manifesting as shared bedrooms and a prohibition against televisions. At least one home was even resistant to installing air conditioning, leaving people who were critically ill stifling in the summer heat.

Though Michael respected Mother Teresa's commitment to care for people in prison or who were infected with HIV, he wanted to create a refuge for his guests. Working with a nearby Catholic parish, Michael built a support network for them. Volunteers helped with household tasks like gardening, giving massages, and driving residents to their doctor appointments. They cooked meals and stopped by to visit. When residents approached their final days, they made sure someone would always be on hand, so no one died alone.

"It's easy to provide food and shelter," Michael recalled, "but it's not easy to provide a safe and clean sanctuary for people who have been rejected and stigmatized. You're not alone when you were born. You shouldn't be alone when you die."

But there were a few rules. He asked the residents to attend weekly meetings so they could talk through inevitable conflicts that arose whenever three strangers share a single home. If the residents had an income, he asked for a donation to help cover the cost of food and utilities—but never more than 30 percent of their already meager earnings. Violence, drugs, and alcohol were prohibited. If someone relapsed, which was bound to happen, Michael helped find a rehabilitation facility to help them get well—and he saved their bedroom until they returned.

True to the Catholic Worker ideals, Michael refused to take government money. He instead relied on donations from the parish, occasional gifts from residents, and even fundraisers hosted by his friend, the spiritual writer Henri Nouwen, a priest who was gay but out only to close friends, who visited to deliver lectures to hundreds of people at San Francisco's Saint Mary's Cathedral and spend time with the guests living at the house.

Over the next few years, more than thirty people lived at Michael's Catholic Worker House. By 1999, when advances in pharmaceutical science meant HIV was no longer a terminal diagnosis, the need for residential hospices lessened and the project ended. But in Michael's view, it had been a success.

Invoking Saint John of the Cross, Michael said the Catholic Worker house had "tried to put love where there had been no love."

———

Hearing about instances of implicit homophobia present in the Catholic Worker movement surprised me, given the reverence many social justice–oriented Catholics hold today for Dorothy Day and the movement she helped launch. When a friend brought me to visit Day's living quarters in New York, I stood in awe while I gazed at the small desk where she wrote. If many Catholics have their way, Day, whose work Pope Francis praised when he spoke to the US Congress in 2015, will be canonized a saint. It's easy to mischaracterize Day decades after her death, as her zeal for the gospel has inspired countless people to engage in social justice activism. And while it's impossible to know how many people with HIV were welcomed by Catholic Workers, at least four other houses of hospitality inspired by Day's example were established in the 1980s and '90s to serve people with AIDS, including Clare House in Cedar Rapids, Iowa, and the Friends of Dorothy House in Syracuse, New York. Day's witness bore fruit, even if it is also true that she was skittish about homosexuality.

The more I reflected on what at first felt like an incongruous reality, I realized that perhaps I shouldn't have been surprised at all. Even today, the most open-minded Catholics can still feel uneasy discussing homosexuality. The church's history of homophobia is long and deep. We can't even seem to agree on how to talk about the issue, much less seek a common destination. And some have simply left the faith, disillusioned with the Church's position.

People like Michael Harank and David Pais certainly offer encouragement, but I know the way they have been able to reconcile their faith and their sexual orientation is remarkable. Both told me simply to ignore homophobic statements and focus instead on the gospel. But many other LGBT Catholics live in a gray zone, where they seem to retain a love for their church but can't quite abide its teachings. As it turned out, another person who inhabits this murkier space lived near me back home in Chicago—someone who, like Michael Harank, had also drawn inspiration from Dorothy Day and the Catholic Worker movement during the height of the AIDS crisis.

———

A newspaper story about an upcoming Chicago election caught my eye. Alderman James Cappleman was up for re-election and a piece of his biographical history intrigued me.

"He came to Chicago in the '80s as a friar with the Franciscans," the article stated. I kept reading. "He eventually left monastic life, came out of the closet, forged a career in social work, and opened a homeless shelter for men dying of AIDS."

The writing made it all sound so linear and simple. Yet deep into my research about AIDS and the Catholic Church at this point, I had so many questions. Why had he joined the Franciscans? What made him leave? Where was the shelter? How did he open it? What role, if any, did his faith play in that work?

A mutual friend volunteered to introduce us. I waited until the election was over (he won) and then asked if he'd be willing to meet for an interview. We planned to talk for about forty-five minutes at his ward office, but I ended up staying for more than two hours.

Stories that touch on themes as complex as spirituality, sexuality, and illness, especially during the height of HIV and AIDS, take many twists and turns. James's stories were no different, his anecdotes filled with overlapping dramas and hesitations about sharing long-buried memories. But one theme spoke to me clearly: He had never been able to separate his faith and his sexual orientation, no matter how persistently he tried.

———

Growing up in a large Catholic family near Houston, Texas, in the 1960s, faith was never far from James's mind. When he was fifteen, his father died by suicide, shattering the family; his mother was left to raise eight children.

About ten months later, Christmas approached. It would be the first holiday season since the loss of their dad for James and his siblings. James's mom refused to let melancholy overtake their lives, instead telling them that they would help another family who was even worse off. That such a family existed was difficult for James to imagine, given the enormity of the loss weighing on him. But his mom worked at a health clinic in Houston, where many patients struggled financially. Everybody seemed to need a little extra assistance at this time of year. The Capplemans loaded up the car with a tree, presents, and the fixings for a complete Christmas dinner and drove out to a family in need. That was a Christmas James would never forget. It showed him that while life was indeed challenging, no matter how trying things might be for you, others had it worse. You needed to do what you could to help. That lesson would stick with him for years.

Later, in his twenties, James taught middle school. He was shocked by the poverty he encountered. He remembers an eleven-year-old girl who was forced into prostitution to help her family afford food. He did what he could to help when he encountered situations like that, but he felt called to a life in which he could do even more. In 1982, he joined a Franciscan religious order, attracted by their namesake, Saint Francis of Assisi, who seemed to reject power and embrace service to the poor. That was what he wanted for himself.

About eleven others joined the community the same year. He enjoyed meeting the other Franciscans, and he found his work fulfilling, ministering at a home for troubled youth and regularly visiting a hospice. Though his entry into religious life seemed to be on track, he still had many questions about his calling.

A group of friars talked one night about HIV and AIDS, many of them expressing a desire to respond to the crisis in concrete ways. Then one friar asked an obvious but difficult question: why were they each so interested in the subject? All but one of the young friars stated that they were gay. Had they not been friars, some wondered, might they also be sick?

Some of the friars had joined the religious order because they were not ready to deal with their sexuality; entering the priesthood provided an easy excuse when it came to questions about dating and marriage. James had known as early as age five that he was different. For a while, he prayed for a cure. He eventually gave up on all that, but that early devotion had helped him develop spiritually, nourishing his call to religious life. All around him, the institutional church was fighting gay rights, but James found his Franciscan community welcoming. He had seemingly reconciled his faith and his sexuality—so why did he feel so restless?

For the next few years, James felt he was constantly bickering with his superiors, whether about the church's views on women or his refusal to wear a Roman collar when he visited patients. It exhausted everyone. Something had to change. He felt called to social work, but his religious superiors had other plans for him. So James called his brother, who happened to be a social worker himself, and explained his predicament.

"You know, if you really want to be a social worker, you need to go for it," his brother told him.

In his mid-thirties, James still wasn't quite ready to go back to school, but he felt in his gut that his brother was right and that his time in the Franciscans was nearing an end. It isn't easy leaving a religious community, which can feel like turning your back on your family, but James knew he was making the right call. He said goodbye and set out on his own path. He was ready to live life as a gay man.

By 1987, James had moved with a boyfriend to Chicago and accepted a teaching job at a Catholic school. Everything seemed to be moving along the right path. Despite their happiness, James and his boyfriend saw young gay men just like them being struck down by AIDS and they wanted to help.

For people living with HIV and AIDS in the 1980s, finding suitable housing could be a major challenge. Non-discrimination laws were rare, and stigma was plentiful. Landlords didn't want to rent to people with AIDS, neighbors didn't want to live near them, and cities often failed to devote enough resources to help. James saw this struggle play out firsthand, when a man his partner knew through work couldn't find housing because of his HIV status. In an effort to help, they turned to friends who ran a Catholic Worker house in Houston to ask for ideas.

"We have room here," the friends offered.

It was hardly an ideal situation, but given the crisis of affordable housing for people with HIV, it seemed the best they could do. The man moved to Houston to live at a Catholic Worker house. But James's friends recognized that this wasn't going to be a permanent solution to the growing challenge of finding housing for people with HIV.

"Chicago should have its own Catholic Worker House, one for people with AIDS," they suggested.

Like Michael Harank in Oakland, both James and his partner had been drawn to the Catholic Worker movement because its founders understood Christianity as a calling to stand with the poor through radical acts of solidarity, far from institutional power and prestige. Why not heed the advice of their friends and open a Chicago-based Catholic Worker House? James and his partner started planning. They raised funds, which included a loan from the Houston Catholic Worker house, and began searching for real estate. They wanted to buy, but that just wasn't realistic with their limited resources. Their initial hunt was frustrating, with landlords refusing to rent once they disclosed who would be living in the units. Eventually, they found a sympathetic building manager and signed a lease for three rental units in a building on Chicago's far north side.

They begged for money and scrounged for used furniture, some of it previously belonging to gay men who died from AIDS and whose families were afraid to touch anything in their homes. They moved everything into the apartment and identified future residents. The Saint Catherine of Genoa Catholic Worker House, named for a sixteenth-century laywoman who ministered to victims of plague, was ready to open.

But there was one problem. There were no holiday decorations and Christmas Day, 1988, was fast approaching. Thinking back to that first Christmas following his father's death, James couldn't let this stand. The guests moving into the apartments deserved holiday cheer as much as anyone else, so a cash-strapped James approached a man at a Christmas tree lot and explained his situation. With Christmas so close, surely the trees wouldn't sell. Plus, it was for a good cause.

"I'm literally begging," James thought, smiling as he recalled the life of Saint Francis. He had never gone without when he was a Franciscan, yet here he was, now living life on his own, pleading for charity.

Successful in his ask, James returned to the apartment. When the residents arrived, they were greeted with a decorated Christmas tree and a pile of presents. Women and babies, the first residents, sat smiling near the tree, with James and his friends on hand to celebrate the holiday.

James felt good about the trajectory of his new life. His vocation as a friar had ended early, but he was grateful for the spiritual discipline he had learned while part of the order. He was now engaged in meaningful work and happily teaching at a Catholic school. His path seemed set. But a short while later, one of James's friends lost his job after a student had spotted him at a Pride parade and reported it. His friend's contract was not renewed.

When James learned what had happened, he was scared. He had told a few close friends that he was gay, but he tried to be discreet. Gays were not allowed to teach at Catholic schools, and he needed to keep his job. If he were fired, his family would want answers, and he wasn't out to them. Maybe working for the church wouldn't work after all.

"You know what kind of people won't care if I'm gay?" he asked himself. "Social workers."

It was time to chase that dream.

James never returned to teaching. While he took classes, he worked part-time at a social service agency, where he helped refugees transition to life in a new country. His Catholic Worker house was filling an important need serving destitute people with AIDS, including women and children. Coming out as gay to more people had instilled in James a sense of freedom previously unknown to him, and he felt an itch to be engaged in the activism world. He attended a meeting of the local ACT UP chapter and decided he would no longer hide. This newfound liberation created some rifts with his partner, and they eventually split. Around the same time, James rethought his relationship with the Catholic Church.

He reflected on statements church leaders made against gay rights, both in Rome and at home in Chicago. He thought the church should do more to help in the fight against HIV and AIDS, or at least stay out of the way of public health experts. He joined Dignity, finding a place to be fully himself while living out his spiritual life. He went on to become a leader in his local chapter.

Over the next few years, James's activism targeted not only civil authorities who weren't doing enough to respond to HIV and AIDS but also Catholics who failed to speak out against hate crimes targeting gay people. In 1992, as president of Dignity's Chicago chapter, he met with Cardinal Bernardin to encourage a stronger institutional voice against gay bashing. Then, he led a contingent to a protest outside the cardinal's mansion, demanding more respect for women and gays in the church. A few years later, in 1996, James was featured in a newspaper story about Dignity's upcoming twenty-fifth anniversary. He's photographed in a coat and tie along with three other gay men sitting in a Methodist church, where Dignity held Masses following its expulsion from Catholic parishes. The article hints at the complicated relationship among the gay Catholics who stayed in Dignity, those who left to join the Archdiocesan Gay and Lesbian Outreach, a church-sanctioned gay and lesbian ministry, and the institutional church itself. James was given the final word about those who sought to hold on to the spiritual gifts of Catholicism while letting go of aspects of the faith that felt harmful to gay and lesbian people.

"This is us creating our own rituals," he said.

———

James left the Saint Catherine of Genoa Catholic Worker House several months after he helped get it off the ground. The house eventually moved, twice, first to an empty convent and then to a rectory attached to a closed parish, both on Chicago's predominantly African American South Side. But by 1997, as protease inhibitor drugs transformed HIV into a chronic but manageable condition, the house was struggling. It received fewer referrals, and widespread drug use among some of the residents who remained in the house made it difficult to form a healthy community. By the end of the summer, the house closed.

People familiar with the history of the Catholic Church in Chicago may be puzzled as to why I profiled this relatively obscure Catholic Worker house. Though it seems to have made strong connections with the local neighborhood, forming partnerships with other Catholic ministries and serving guests for about a decade, it seems not to have evolved into a major resource for the city. In fact, there was a much larger AIDS hospice founded in 1989 by a Catholic religious order called Bonaventure House, which still operates today. Cardinal Joseph Bernardin had pledged $200,000 and the Alexian Brothers promised half a million dollars more toward the project, which at the time doubled the number of available beds for people with AIDS in need of hospice help, all carried out over the objections of neighbors. Bonaventure House is an excellent example of the institutional church's pastoral response to HIV and AIDS, and, in fact, Sister Carol and Sister Mary Ellen visited it at one point to learn more about HIV and AIDS ministry.

But James's place in all this history has stuck with me, because it encapsulates the messy reality of what it means to be gay and Catholic. He was attracted to religious life until he wasn't. He's had complicated relationships with church authorities. In 1991, he met his partner at church and more than two decades later, they consecrated their relationship with a blessing from a Catholic woman fighting for the right to be ordained as a priest. James is not sure he's Catholic today, though he still attends Dignity Masses, which are still held in a Protestant church in Boystown. Dignity's relationship with the institutional church is even more complicated, but its members still fight for LGBT inclusion.

There isn't a single way, I've learned, to integrate the complex reality of living as both gay and Catholic. David Pais grew angry at the church but fought his way back in. Michael Harank focused on the gospel and ignored the hierarchy, finding communities that accepted him for who he was. James Cappleman, and countless other LGBT Catholics, live somewhere in the middle.

14

A TANGIBLE LOVE

Father Bill McNichols jumped on the subway and zigzagged his way through New York City. He had to get up to the Bronx, where a young man lay dying at home, then back downtown to Saint Vincent's for his regular rounds. He would have to take the train out to New Jersey later that night. He felt like he might collapse from the strain of trying to keep up. So many people asked for his time, and perhaps influenced by a new form of worship becoming popular in some Christian circles, they also asked him deliver healing.

Father Bill was somewhat wary of the healing movement that became popular in the 1970s and 80s. There were too many charlatans on television promising physical health in exchange for cash. Bill wanted nothing to do with that. "It's messy. There's all kinds of hysteria and fanaticism," he thought.

But Father Bill listened to people who expressed a desire for a more nuanced form of healing. Their requests seemed reasonable. They sought physical healing, of course. Who didn't? But if that wasn't in the cards, they wanted to be at peace with whatever awaited them on the other side. He could get behind that.

For inspiration, Father Bill sought advice from a Catholic nun who organized healing services. He wanted to learn how to listen more intensely to the sick, how to ask about their concerns gently, and then how to pray that God would offer healing that was physical, emotional, and spiritual. He was eager to explore how this kind of prayer could be incorporated into his HIV and AIDS ministry.

When asked to explain the role prayer played in his work, Father Bill put it like this: "I speak very simply to God. I say, 'Look, help this person.' I have no control over God, whether he answers." But as more people turned to him for spiritual care, he realized there were more requests than hours in the day. He wanted to help everyone in need, but it became clear that individual visits were not enough. He had to find a way to minister to more people at once.

On a walk through the city, Father Bill passed by a church on Fourteenth Street, Our Lady of Guadalupe. He knew the church well, since two of his personal heroes, the Catholic Worker founder Dorothy Day and the peace activist Thomas Merton, had worshipped there. Father Bill, thinking how best to minister to a growing list of people affected by HIV and AIDS, was inspired. He wondered if the priests who ran the church would allow him to host a healing Mass there, a prime spot given its location near New York's large gay community. He stepped inside, said a prayer, then asked for permission to use the space.

"You can use the church," the priest told Father Bill. But with one condition: he couldn't promote the Masses too widely.

That conditional offer might have discouraged or angered other people. In the late 1980s, there was so much stigma around AIDS. But Father Bill understood that even some ministers who served people with AIDS were reluctant to talk openly about their work. The priest's trepidation made sense. Given the fear around the disease, would the church's regular worshippers be uncomfortable gathering in a building that had been used days earlier for an AIDS Mass? No matter how often you told people they simply could not contract HIV by sitting on the same bench as someone who had AIDS, or even by hugging or shaking hands, the fear could be overwhelming. So Father Bill didn't dwell on the request. Instead, he rejoiced that he had found a space to offer healing Masses. Then he got to planning.

He reached out to like-minded priests and nuns to help spread word of the Masses. If someone approached them for spiritual support, Father Bill asked, would they please send them to the healing Mass? Word got around and about one hundred people showed up for the first Mass. Father Bill was moved by the crowd. So much unmet need.

During Mass, he asked the congregation to say aloud the names of people who needed their prayers, perhaps those who were sick or who had died from AIDS. Voices filled the church in a dizzying chorus of anguish. At the end of Mass, Father Bill changed out of his vestments and into a sweater and a pair of corduroys. Two lay women active in the healing movement joined him at the front of the church. One by one, those in attendance approached the three ministers and asked for prayers.

"What is it you want from God?" Father Bill asked as each person approached.

The responses ranged from requests for immediate physical healing to more cerebral and spiritual concerns. Some were desperate for relief from the harsh physical symptoms associated with AIDS, an end to diarrhea, headaches, weakness, and night sweats. Others, perhaps more skeptical of divine intervention for medical realities, asked Father Bill to pray for spiritual and emotional healing.

"I'd like to be less terrified."

"I'd like to feel better."

"Help me find hope."

Some people were too ill to sit upright during Mass, so they lay down in the pew. When it came time to approach Father Bill for prayers, they dug deep, mustering up as much energy as possible and leaning on friends and loved ones to make their way toward the altar. If they had enough strength left in them to speak, they voiced aloud what they sought. But some were too weak. They stood silently in front of Father Bill, who prayed over them, asking God for healing. For many, it was the last time they saw Father Bill in this life. He would celebrate their funeral Masses in the weeks and months to come. For others, the experience could be life-giving.

At one of the Masses, a twenty-eight-year-old gay man walked to the front of the church. He had learned a few months earlier that he was HIV-positive. Back home in DC, he and his partner adjusted to life with HIV, throwing themselves into service to others. But tonight, at Mass, the young man, an Episcopalian active in AIDS activism, focused on his own health, asking for "an opening to the healing of positive force." He sobbed during the prayers, finding release and affirmation, recognizing that he was not alone.

Another attendee was struck by the power the prayers offered the sick. The Masses lasted for hours, the church sweltering in the summer heat. The line for blessings was long but those gathered waited patiently.

"At Father Bill's Mass, people could bring their pain and sorrow to Christ and to the Christian community and experience God's saving grace," the attendee observed. "He is the most Christ-like man I have ever met."

———

David Pais had heard about Father Bill's healing Masses. Less than two years after his own HIV diagnosis, his partner, also named Bill, was now very sick. David had relied on his faith to help him accept these challenges. When he read about a healing Mass at a Catholic parish near Chelsea, he thought of his partner. At this point, a nurse was stationed in David and Bill's shared apartment. One evening, David told the nurse that he would be away for a little while. Before David left, he held his partner.

There wasn't much David could do for his partner at this point except pray.

"I'm going to a healing Mass and I'm going to ask the priest for a special blessing for you," David said. "I'll be back in about an hour."

He went to church.

Mass comforted David: the ritual was familiar, the candlelight gentle. Plus, seeing so many others struggling with the senselessness of AIDS offered a feeling of solidarity. Some people climbed the stairs with the help of crutches. Others no longer tried to hide the purple lesions covering their necks and arms. David felt he was in a holy space, a refuge for those cast aside by the world. He closed his eyes, prayed, and wept.

At the end of Mass, David approached Father Bill.

"I think my partner is in his last stages and I'd like to ask you for some kind of message."

Father Bill listened to David's request, and then he prayed. His mind transported him back home to the Southwest, where he remembered a custom in cemeteries in which friends and family of the deceased place candles inside wax paper bags. Lights to guide their loved ones home. Father Bill was moved by the memory, and he told David, "When you go home tonight, tell Bill that the Blessed Virgin Mary is setting up luminaria to guide him home."

Back home, David climbed into bed next to his partner. He whispered Father Bill's message, promising him he wouldn't be alone on the next journey.

A few hours later, Bill died. David envisioned the candles, the luminaria, guiding Bill home, making it easier for him to find his way to peace. Father Bill's image brought comfort to David when he felt his world was falling apart.

"Even as he was dying, I was so grateful for God bringing him into my life," David recalled. "God was never more tangible than my love and attention and service to Bill."

———

Following the death of his partner, and then Dignity's expulsion from Saint Francis Xavier, David was angry and stopped attending church. But in 1994, having moved back to New York after seven years away, he asked a Protestant friend for a recommendation as to where he might find a church that affirmed gay and lesbian believers. David said he longed for spiritual nourishment, a renewed connection to the sacraments that had once been so meaningful to him as a younger man.

"David," his friend told him, smiling, "I cannot recommend an Episcopal parish to you. You are hopelessly Catholic."

When his friend suggested that David visit Saint Francis Xavier, because he had heard good things about their LGBT ministry, David froze. So much emotion packed into that single building. But he told his friend he would try.

Two weeks later, on a warm Sunday in August, he followed through. He climbed once again the stone steps and entered a church that he had once described as his spiritual home. But he felt like an unwelcome outsider that day. He wanted to sit close to the door so that should he hear a single homophobic remark, he could bolt. He chose a pew in the very back of the church.

At the end of Mass, David was in tears. He felt he was finally back home.

When I visited Saint Francis Xavier in 2019, I was struck by its grand scale, elaborate paintings of the stations of the cross, and colorful, antique Tiffany windows. But one of David's favorite details about his parish is at the front of the church.

The parish completed a restoration in 2010 and the original oak kneelers dating back to 1882 had been removed from the pews. They were fashioned into an altar, placed prominently in the sanctuary today. The prayers of generations of Catholics, including untold numbers of souls whose lives were affected in unknown ways by HIV and AIDS, are represented in that altar, petitions and thanksgivings and lamentations. David sees the wood from the kneelers on which he had prayed when Bill was dying, when he grappled with his own HIV diagnosis, when he had lost dozens of friends to AIDS, and at a Mass when he had mourned being ejected from his spiritual home.

"Now, all those prayers are congregated in that altar," David told me.

He said he often thinks of the many Catholics he knew who had been engaged in the fight for justice in the church, as well as his friends who had left the faith, but whose early exposure to the gospel prompted them to demand better treatment for people with HIV.

"Many of the people who were doing that work are gone now, so they are part of my litany of the saints that continue to inspire me to do this work," he said.

Today, David again prays regularly inside Saint Francis Xavier, where he chooses a seat in the front pew.

15

REDEEMED IN SAN FRANCISCO

On a beautiful November evening a few years ago, I found myself attending a reception inside an ornate Vatican museum. I scanned the room, looking for familiar faces so I didn't have to stand awkwardly alone. Cocktail parties filled exclusively with strangers rank among the least enjoyable experiences I can imagine. But I caught sight of an old man whose face I recognized from my research, so I mustered up the courage to introduce myself.

"Hi, Archbishop Quinn," I said. "I'm a journalist, and I'm working on a project about the Catholic Church's early response to the HIV and AIDS crisis."

John R. Quinn was appointed to lead the Archdiocese of San Francisco in 1977 and he held that post until his retirement in 1995. For nearly two decades, he had led Catholics in one of the cities hardest hit by AIDS during the worst years of the epidemic.

The archbishop, in his eighties when we met, took a second to gauge what I was saying. He asked me to explain more. I told him that the goal of my project was to document stories about how Catholics responded to HIV and AIDS, often under the radar, stories that risked being lost forever if they weren't captured soon. His eyes widened. This was in many ways ancient history.

"Yes, there are so many stories," he replied, a note of sadness in his voice. "So many young people died."

He told me about one moment, fairly early in the crisis, that helped shift his view about how the church should respond. A young man, twenty-two, who was living in San Francisco, began feeling sick. When he learned that he had contracted HIV, he considered his life up to that point. He was not yet out to his family, but he wanted his mother to know the truth, so he told her he was gay and tried to steel her for the battle ahead. He hoped the revelation would help bring them closer. He was wrong.

"Twenty-two years ago, my only mistake," the mother said, wrapping her arm around her son, "was not having an abortion."

The archbishop was silent for a moment.

"It was just awful," he said. "And there are so many other stories."

The room was noisy, the sound of celebration at odds with the heaviness of our conversation, and I didn't want to take up more of his time. He mentioned that there were many people in San Francisco who had other memories to share, and he offered to talk more once we both returned home.

But a few days after our conversation, I heard that the archbishop had suffered a fall in Rome. The outlook wasn't good. He had been admitted to a hospital. That June, about six months after our brief conversation, he died. Our formal interview never materialized. A man who held a front-row seat to one of recent history's most difficult moments was now gone. And with him, so many untold stories. Archbishop Quinn's death renewed my sense of urgency that this project had to be completed soon or many more stories would vanish. I knew then that I had no choice but to board a plane. My destination was a Catholic parish in the middle of San Francisco's gay neighborhood, the Castro, that had faced a stark choice in the early days of the AIDS epidemic: respond with mercy or get out of the way.

———

Back in the day, Christmas meant the world to the parishioners of Most Holy Redeemer Parish, the church covered in greenery, candlelight bouncing off the stained-glass windows. At the center of it all was the crèche, the baby Jesus reminding those gathered near the church that a bit of heaven existed right there in San Francisco's Eureka Valley. Young families packed into the church for Mass, singing familiar hymns and reveling in the season. But by the end of the 1970s, those days were long gone, with nearly all the working-class Catholic families leaving San Francisco for the suburbs. Most Holy Redeemer was now a shell of its former self, with just a few old timers sticking around. The parish's future, if it had one, looked bleak.

The Castro, the area immediately surrounding the parish, was under going a transformation. By 1980, large numbers of young gay men had moved in, opening bars and bookstores and creating an accepting community. The sidewalks bustled with energy, a youthful vibe seemingly everywhere. Except at Most Holy Redeemer.

With the limitless possibilities for gay and lesbian people in the Castro, it seemed almost unforgivable to have a church in the middle of it all that felt so moribund. Surely the parish could be a welcoming space and harness some of the neighborhood's renewed creative spirit? A group of young gay Catholics seemed to think so.

I visited Most Holy Redeemer in the fall of 2019, finally checking off a key destination on my gay Catholic pilgrimage bucket list. Many

Catholics had told me about the LGBT ministry there, but I had never managed to make it to the parish during previous trips to California. The morning of my visit, I took the train and laughed as I ascended on the escalator at Castro Station. Rainbow lights bounced off the shiny surfaces, creating a clublike vibe even on public transit. The sun was shining, and the Castro brimmed with people. I walked a few blocks and found Tom Battipaglia, my guide for the afternoon. Tom joined Most Holy Redeemer back in the early 1990s and he had agreed to give me a walking tour of the Castro. I had been to the neighborhood before, but I wanted the local perspective from somebody who could help me understand life here in the 1980s and 90s.

As we walked, Tom joked that the Castro today wasn't much like it had been back then. With its rainbow crosswalks and escalators, it's now "more like gay Disneyland," as he put it. But history is everywhere. He told me about the good times, when he moved here from New York and felt like the world was his for the taking. San Francisco was a dream destination for a young, attractive kid like him. He worked in a couple of bars, made great friends. But then word traveled through the community that previously healthy gay men were getting sick. Before he knew it, his friends were dying. He eventually tested positive for HIV himself. As we continued to walk, the past came to life. He teared up thinking of the friends he had lost to AIDS.

There was a brighter spot in the otherwise overwhelmingly dark memories. Tom said that finding a community of gay men at Most Holy Redeemer—some of whom were like him, living with HIV and AIDS— saved his life. After the tour, I thanked Tom and we went our separate ways. I absorbed the energy of the neighborhood today from a nearby coffee shop. Small groups of gay men walked by, some pairs holding hands, but mixed in were straight couples, some pushing strollers. Like many gay neighborhoods, the Castro faces an unknown future. But I was curious to learn more about its past, so I packed up my laptop and headed to the church.

———

Father Tony McGuire arrived at the sleepy parish in 1982. He didn't know much about the church, other than a general impression that it was "on the skids." The young families had left first, followed in short order by the nuns who had staffed the now shuttered school. Their empty convent across the street seemed to underline just how far the parish had fallen. Father Tony's task was to bring life back to Most Holy Redeemer.

He started by taking stock of who attended Mass each week. The small crowd was mostly elderly, people who had lived in the neighborhood for decades and were still loyal to the parish. But he also noticed a handful of young men who popped in for Mass but who weren't too involved in any other part of parish life. As Father Tony put it, he realized pretty quickly that Most Holy Redeemer served the "gays and the grays."

The grays knew the parish's history and stood by the church even as its membership deteriorated. They represented the past, but Father Tony thought they deserved a vibrant community in their twilight. The gays seemed committed to their faith, choosing to attend Mass even as the Church made life difficult for gay Catholics. They represented the future of the parish. Father Tony suspected it would take the gays and the grays working together to save this church.

Given Most Holy Redeemer's reputation today as a bright spot for LGBT ministry in the Catholic Church, I was surprised to learn that there were several bumps in the beginning. Early in Father Tony's tenure at the church, members of Most Holy Redeemer invited the San Francisco chapter of Dignity to move its weekly Mass to the parish. The invitation made sense, given the church's prime location in the Castro and the fact that Most Holy Redeemer didn't offer an LGBT ministry. But Father Tony was leery of the proposal. He thought parishes should serve their neighborhoods, an aspiration Most Holy Redeemer clearly failed to meet given the parish's small and relatively inactive gay membership. He feared that welcoming Dignity would segregate the gays from the grays and thwart his vision of the two communities relying on one another for spiritual support. So in December 1983, Father Tony rescinded the invitation, for one year, to buy time for his experiment.

Some gay activists were furious.

"After denying Dignity, the gay Catholic organization, the use of your church (even though it is as much theirs as yours—as only God is the landlord), it is but the next step to close down any outreach to Gay and Lesbian Catholics," read an editor's note in the *Bay Area Reporter*, a local gay newspaper, accusing Father Tony of wanting to end gay outreach altogether. The note zeroed in on Most Holy Redeemer's demographic challenges, writing, "Of course, there's always the fear that Gays attending your services at Holy Redeemer might contaminate your rapidly aging and declining congregation. It will then join the ranks of one more sacrosanct but empty Catholic church."

Having angered the gay community, it was on Father Tony to prove his sincerity in his desire to welcome gay and lesbian Catholics back to church—a task made more difficult by broader church politics.

———

Following the murder of gay civil rights activist Harvey Milk in 1978, many in San Francisco's gay and lesbian community felt emboldened, like they were on the edge of a new era. Gay and lesbian Catholics in the Bay Area, like elsewhere, were no less vocal about demanding a place in the church, leading to conflict with church leaders.

Around this time, many gay Catholics viewed Archbishop Quinn with disdain. He had disbanded an archdiocesan task force addressing gay and lesbian issues because some members had questioned the church's ban on homosexual sex. Shortly after, he became embroiled in a controversy over a gay domestic partnership measure under consideration by the Board of Supervisors.

Gay activists said the bill was especially important because it would allow an individual to stay on their same-sex partner's health insurance if they became sick, a crucial human right in the era of AIDS. The bill passed the city's Board of Supervisors, but Mayor Dianne Feinstein signaled publicly that she was unsure if she supported it. Sensing an opportunity to kill the bill, the archbishop urged her to exercise her veto power, warning in a letter that the law would "further erode the moral foundations of civilized society" by equating gay relationships with marriage. The archbishop's spokesman articulated the dynamics more crudely, telling reporters that while the church's opposition to the bill was not meant to be an attack on gay people, "we can't go along with equating shacking up with marriage." Gay Catholics felt betrayed when the mayor vetoed the measure, in line with the archdiocese's wishes, and accused Archbishop Quinn of being blind to the needs of his flock.

Against this turmoil between the gay community and the archdiocese, Father Tony tried to undertake steps to transform the parish. There were early signs it wouldn't be easy. Some of the grays at Most Holy Redeemer didn't want to welcome gay Catholics into their church, particularly after a ribald party in the parish hall pushed the levels of their tolerance. Shortly after Father Tony arrived, a former Catholic asked him if his AA group could use the parish hall for a Halloween party. Father Tony said yes, hoping that perhaps the welcoming gesture would be a sign of goodwill between the parish and the gay community. But Father Tony was new to the Castro. He didn't know that Halloween there was a wild affair, filled with elaborate costumes, often with little clothing involved. Though this Halloween party took place in a church, the salaciousness of a Castro Halloween knew no boundaries. Drag queens were dressed to the nines and told bawdy jokes. Men donned risqué costumes and bared lots of skin. One of the grays took notice, and she was not happy.

"It was like Sodom and Gomorrah!" she yelled at Father Tony.

Father Tony zinged back, "Well, maybe Sodom!"

As for the gays, Father Tony recognized their anger over Archbishop Quinn's stance on civil rights and their disappointment stemming from his own decision regarding Dignity. He hoped a listening session might alleviate some of the tension, so he invited parishioners to a social gathering outside Mass. About a dozen people showed up, a mixture of the gays and the grays. Just what Father Tony wanted. He invited them to share their experiences of belonging to the church and asked them to describe their ideal parish. One of the gay men talked about how difficult it was to reconcile his Catholic faith with his sexuality. A gray highlighted her struggles as a widow belonging to a parish where so much social life had revolved around family. Father Tony said he could empathize with their struggles, as his vow of celibacy contributed to a sense of loneliness. The shared vulnerability created a mutual trust among the gays and the grays. Though it was just one step, and a small one at that, Father Tony was encouraged. But there was more work to do if gay Catholics were to feel truly welcome at Most Holy Redeemer.

———

As the 1980s wore on and HIV and AIDS affected more people in the Castro, a small group of gays who belonged to Most Holy Redeemer suggested that their parish had a moral obligation to respond. When I visited, I met with as many of these parish organizers as I could find. They're all a bit older now, but back in the 1980s, they would have been in their twenties and thirties, young gay Catholics unwilling to be denied a place in their church.

I took the train to Oakland to meet Cliff Morrison, a retired nurse whose determination to open an AIDS ward at San Francisco General Hospital is well known thanks to the 2018 documentary film *5B*. What isn't as widely recognized is how he leaned on his Catholic faith during those horrible early days of AIDS and how he helped transform Most Holy Redeemer.

Cliff moved from his home in Florida to San Francisco in 1979, drawn to the city's gay scene and the freedom it represented. He felt like a kid in a candy store. His friends teased him for being something of a prude, since he didn't drink too much and he found the party scene unappealing. But after a childhood of feeling that life as a gay man would be sorrowful and lonely, he was thrilled finally to be surrounded by other young gay men. As he settled into his new life, he sought out a spiritual home. He was delighted during a stroll through the Castro when, near the gay bars and bookstores, he stumbled on a Catholic church.

Cliff attended Mass one Sunday and was somewhat dismayed by what he saw. The crowd was sparse, with mostly elderly parishioners. Maybe his dream, a Catholic parish in the Castro catering to the gay community, was too good to be true. But he decided to keep going to Mass anyway. He eventually invited a few gay friends. Then he hung flyers around the Castro and urged Father Tony to place ads in gay newspapers.

Some of the grays fled Most Holy Redeemer in the early days of Father Tony's project, when people like Cliff and his friends became more visible in the parish. But a few hung on. Unfortunately, since so much time has passed since the 1980s, I wasn't able to meet any of the original grays. In fact, some of the grays at the parish today started out as gays at the start of this history. So I asked the gays I met if they remembered any of the grays, and more than a few mentioned one particular woman.

Marie Krystoflak was a grandmother who had spent much of her life active at Most Holy Redeemer, who could easily remember brighter days when the church was filled with families and social activities. She had lamented the parish's decline but was encouraged when she saw Sunday Mass taking on a more youthful energy with the increasing numbers of gay men joining. Rather than flee like some of the other grays, she stood outside the front doors on the steps, welcoming the young men to church. She learned their names. Asked how their week had gone. If she hadn't seen them at Mass, she approached them the following Sunday, curious why they had missed church. Week by week, Marie bridged the space between the gays and the grays.

As Christmas approached one year, Cliff met with Father Tony. The Castro took festivities seriously, and Christmas was no different: The entire neighborhood celebrated the season with lights, garlands, trees, and wreaths. They were everywhere, it seemed, though Most Holy Redeemer felt dead. Cliff told Father Tony this presented an opportunity.

"Most of these guys, they moved here from the Midwest and the South, and a lot of them are Catholic. Why don't we invite them back?"

A team of parishioners created the "Come Home for Christmas" campaign. They hung flyers and banners. They strung greenery at the church. They ordered candles, so many candles. And at the center of it all, situated outside so the entire neighborhood could enjoy it, stood a crèche. Christmas had returned to Most Holy Redeemer. All they needed now were worshippers.

Cliff and the other gays were proven right. More than a few gays came home for Christmas. Some of the grays still weren't sure what to make of the new crowd. But that there was a crowd at all showed that life could return to the parish. The joy of Christmas was back for one more year. But soon, the parish was called on to provide more than Christmas cheer.

———

By the mid-1980s, the Castro was heavily affected by the rising death toll from AIDS. The local pharmacy posted photos of limbs covered in the purple KS lesions, a warning to others about the deadly disease. The neighborhood was on edge, and Most Holy Redeemer was no exception.

At this point, parish ministry had been thriving for a couple of years. With AIDS progressing, dozens of parishioners met in the empty parish convent across the street, intent on figuring out how best to respond. During those meetings, it became clear that there were not enough outlets for people to find emotional and spiritual support. Stigma around HIV and AIDS was strong, even in the Castro, and spaces to talk freely were sparse. The parish had both space and a supportive community. An idea was born.

Cliff Morrison was now a full-time nurse at San Francisco General Hospital. He worked around the clock opening the AIDS ward, but he also managed to carve out time to attend Mass. When he saw that the parish was serious about responding to AIDS, he stepped up. He knew that education about HIV was critical in combatting its spread, so he hosted a workshop at the parish for people who wanted to volunteer. He taught the basics, like the difference between HIV and AIDS and how the virus was not easily transferable. Most of all, Cliff told his fellow parishioners about the importance of listening empathetically to people with AIDS, rather than making assumptions about what they needed.

With their training complete, parishioners set up a neighborhood buddy program to help with everyday tasks like laundry and cooking. Most of the volunteers were parishioners already involved with the budding AIDS ministry, but the program needed more people to respond to the growing need. When parish leaders asked the gays for help, many simply couldn't change their work schedules. But what about the grays? They were retired and certainly had time. And many of the widows were pretty good cooks. Would they be willing to help a community whose lives seemed so different from their own?

Many of the Irish and Italian grandmothers who had stuck around during the lean years at Most Holy Redeemer, to then revel in the renewed community created by the influx of gay men, responded with gusto when they saw the great need that resulted from AIDS. The grays cooked meals. They dropped off food. They sat and listened.

Across the street from the church sat the now empty convent, which had hosted the early gatherings of what grew into the parish's AIDS ministry, which by now was well on its way toward becoming a neighborhood institution. From those early meetings sprang an AIDS support group, the buddy program, and occasional educational events. But some of the parishioners realized that many people with AIDS had no suitable place to live after they became sick. A local group approached the parish with an idea: why not transform the empty convent into a hospice? Father Tony and many parishioners supported the idea, and plans barreled ahead. The archdiocese agreed to lease the building to the hospice. But there was still one catch: the parish didn't have enough money to donate to fully fund the venture. That's when a decidedly Catholic solution was born.

Each Thursday night, gays and grays from the parish, plus friends from the Castro, gathered at the parish for lively games of bingo. Local businesses donated prizes and the proceeds benefited what would become the Coming Home Hospice. Bingo alone attracted people all over the city, but bingo in the Castro meant the presence of attractive young men who could lure in the masses. One volunteer flitted through the crowd, using his "green eyes [and] a smile that won't stop" to sell raffle tickets and rake in the cash. It was, after all, for a good cause.

Though the hospice operated independently of the church, many parishioners, including Marie Krystoflak, volunteered. The plight of the young men she saw each time she stopped by weighed heavily on her. "By the grace of God, they could be one of my children," Marie thought, picturing the two sons she had brought to Most Holy Redeemer when they were young. "What the straight people have to do, and I'm straight, is to learn to have a little compassion and understanding. We can't point the finger at anybody, because God will judge us one day." Marie became a regular at the bingo games, serving up drinks and snacks to the players. And once again, helped bring together the two communities.

The combination of gays and grays and bingo worked. The games eventually raised more than $140,000 for the hospice.

———

The support group, buddy program, and hospice were vital assets to the Castro. But Most Holy Redeemer was above all a church, a place for people to gather for prayer and worship. And those gatherings became increasingly gay. Attendance at Sunday Mass had doubled since Father Tony's arrival, with more than half the congregation now gay men. In the era of AIDS, that sadly meant funerals were increasing as well, quadrupling in just three years. Some parishioners recognized the spiritual component of any terminal illness and the lack of pastoral resources available for people with AIDS. They wanted to ensure the parish responded to the epidemic spiritually. Each week, Father Tony prayed by name for parishioners who were sick. And each week, the list of previously healthy young men grew longer.

One of the grays had been moved by the growing list of names and approached Father Tony with a question: "Whatever happened to Forty Hours?"

The Forty Hours Devotion had long ago been a mainstay in some parishes, with Catholics taking turns gathering inside a church to pray in front of the consecrated host, the body of Christ, for forty hours straight. But following the reforms of the Second Vatican Council, the practice had fallen out of favor.

In answering the question, Father Tony said he wasn't entirely sure of the devotion's history, but he believed it started back in 1537 as a plea for God's mercy as a plague tore through Milan.

"Don't we have a plague here?"

It was true. At this point, AIDS killed about forty people each month in San Francisco. Even if his memory wasn't exactly right—Forty Hours had actually started as a wartime prayer—resurrecting the devotion to combat the growing threat seemed worthwhile.

That August, over the course of forty hours, hundreds of people packed into Most Holy Redeemer. They worshipped at Mass, prayed for healing, meditated on suffering, and adored the Eucharist. Archbishop Quinn's reputation with the gay community had healed a bit since his opposition to the gay rights bill, but he still had much to learn about the struggles of gay Catholics. He visited the parish during the Forty Hours, anointing those who were sick. He asked questions about the Coming Home Hospice. On Sunday morning, he was back at Most Holy Redeemer, celebrating Mass for six hundred people gathered inside the church.

By the end of the weekend, Archbishop Quinn experienced something of an epiphany about AIDS, listening to people whose lives had been changed by the disease. He still had work to do to gain the trust of the gay community. Following the service, the local gay paper reported on the event, and faulted Archbishop Quinn for not saying "AIDS" or "gay" during the service and noted that Dignity, still angry over Father Tony's rescinded invitation, was unimpressed with the vigil, since its members had already been engaged in AIDS ministry. But over the next few years, Archbishop Quinn continued visiting the parish, meeting members of the gay community and learning firsthand about their fears, struggles, joys, and talents.

A few months before the Vatican released its incendiary letter on homosexuality, in 1986, Archbishop Quinn wrote an essay about ministry to people with AIDS. A sign of his comfort was his use of the colloquial term "gay" rather than the more clinical-sounding "homosexual." He commended a gay man for showing compassion and care to his dying partner and he condemned those who preached that AIDS was divine retribution.

Archbishop Quinn's increased understanding of the impact of AIDS on the gay community prompted him to persuade other senior church leaders to take the crisis more seriously—including those at the Vatican.

Ahead of Pope John Paul II's visit to the United States in 1987, which was to include a stop in San Francisco, Archbishop Quinn flew to Rome to meet with the pope. During a private meeting, he urged the pope to meet people with AIDS during his trip. I was stunned to learn that even by 1987, when AIDS was a global crisis and a year after the Vatican released its letter condemning homosexuality, the widely revered Pope John Paul II still had not made a formal statement about HIV and AIDS. Archbishop Quinn seemed to find this objectionable.

"AIDS is such a prominent feature of life for so many people in San Francisco, for people who have the disease, their families, and their friends," he said of his plea for the pope to meet with people with AIDS. "I thought it would be appropriate for the pope to show some gesture of concern and compassion in that direction."

The Vatican agreed to Archbishop Quinn's request. Initial plans were even floated for the pope to visit the Coming Home Hospice, which would have elevated the profile of Most Holy Redeemer and bestowed an honor on the hard work of the gays and the grays to form an integrated parish. But while gay Catholics in San Francisco were coming around to their archbishop, the church still had work to do with the gay community as a whole. Suggesting the pope drop by the Castro set off a flurry of objections.

The Sisters of Perpetual Indulgence, gay activists who dressed as nuns, protested Archbishop Quinn. Like ACT UP, they believed the church's teaching against condoms harmed the gay community's fight against

HIV. Many Catholics found the bawdy representation of nuns offensive. But some of the drag performers who comprised the group said they were actually paying homage to Catholic sisters, the women who historically worked in the trenches.

One member of the group, Sister Boom Boom, whose real name was Jack Fertig, actually became Catholic after taking classes at Most Holy Redeemer. Although Sister Boom Boom was a gay activist who mocked nuns, he said that becoming Catholic was not a denunciation of his sexuality.

"Sister never batted an eyelash," Jack Fertig said of the sister who led the classes at the parish, "but asked if I could show up Sunday mornings at eight."

Despite that relative calm between the local church and the gay community in San Francisco—there were still occasional clashes—gay activists were still angry at the Vatican for its anti-gay views. They resented the idea of Pope John Paul II visiting the Castro for what they said was a photo op. Sensing that the event might prompt protest, the Vatican changed its plans. When the pope arrived in San Francisco, he visited another church, where he greeted a group of people with AIDS, including two priests. (Scrapping plans for John Paul II to visit the Castro hardly meant the papal visit was free of controversy. Demonstrators greeted the pope in San Francisco after a top Vatican official, the American Archbishop John Foley, told a reporter just ahead of the pope's arrival that gay men contracted AIDS "because they engaged in what we would consider to be objectively immoral behavior." John Paul II himself deflected when a reporter asked him on their flight to the United States if AIDS was a punishment from God, stating, "It's not easy to know the intentions of God Himself. He is a great mystery. We know that he is justice, mercy, and love.")

Overall, the vitriol between gay activists and the church in San Francisco never seemed to reach the same levels of hostility as it had in New

York. Archbishop Quinn took a more conciliatory tone with gay activists than Cardinal O'Connor had in New York, perhaps easing some of the tension in the process. During the pope's visit, Quinn had served as something of an unlikely bridge between rightward-slanting Vatican officials and Catholic liberals in San Francisco. After the papal visit that he had helped plan, Quinn continued his outreach to gay and lesbian Catholics. There were hiccups along the way, including when he again opposed same-sex spousal rights in 1989. But the archbishop credited meeting gay and lesbian people in person, often at Most Holy Redeemer, as driving his pastoral response.

"Through personal contact," Archbishop Quinn said, "[gay people] have ceased to be abstractions that you read about in a book. They are people. You see the problems and sufferings they have to experience. I feel I have grown in understanding through those experiences."

———

Father Tony McGuire's experiment back in 1982 wasn't aimed at convincing an archbishop to show greater understanding to gay Catholics. Nor was it necessarily to create vital community resources like support groups or hospices. Instead, he wanted Most Holy Redeemer to be a spiritual home to the people who lived their lives in the Castro. One interview in particular suggests that Father Tony succeeded.

I met Thomas Ellerby in the rectory at Most Holy Redeemer. The high cost of living in San Francisco had prompted him to move out to Oakland, so he hadn't visited the parish in several years. But back in the 1980s, someone mentioned to him that he should check out this "gay church in the Castro." Thomas had his issues with the Catholic Church. Though he had been raised in the faith and loved going to Mass, he resented the homophobia he felt permeating the church. But as soon as he arrived at Most Holy Redeemer, he experienced something different.

After Thomas was diagnosed with HIV in 1989, at just twenty-five years old, he was relieved that Most Holy Redeemer had a community in place to support him. He signed up for the "buddy program" when he became too sick to cook meals or do laundry. What he really wanted from his buddy, though, was someone to talk about faith and spirituality. The buddy assigned to him was a straight Catholic woman, Clotilde, and they became fast friends. They attended the parish's Christmas parties together, elaborate affairs with ice sculptures, piles of decadent canapés, and—since Most Holy Redeemer was in the Castro—a fair share of drag queens.

"That was the most fantastic escape from what was going on around us," Thomas told me.

Escaping the reality of AIDS, even if only temporarily, was important to Thomas. As he put it, he faced many hardships outside the walls of Most Holy Redeemer. "One, I was Black. Two, I was gay. Three, I had AIDS. So there was a lot of discrimination to go around."

What kept him going, as he struggled with the death all around him, with his own failing health, and with the racial discrimination he faced in the Castro, was his Catholic faith—lived out in the community at Most Holy Redeemer.

As for Father Tony's vision, Thomas told me that in some ways, it was easy for him to describe the parish to someone like me who wasn't around in those dark early years of AIDS.

"They served the community," he said. "It just so happened to be a gay community, that was ground zero for HIV and AIDS. The parish was in the business of saving souls and saving lives."

———

Back at the parish, I walked around the grounds trying to fill time before my interviews. I noticed a couple of glassed-in bulletin boards outside.

They contained flyers covered in rainbows. One said, "God's inclusive love is proclaimed here." Another depicted an upside-down pink triangle. Written in big block letters, the flyer read, "Stop the Violence. Safe place." I had noticed them posted on windows of gay bars, bookstores, and cafés throughout the Castro. It was heartening to see one displayed at a Catholic church.

A statue of the Virgin Mary caught my eye in the courtyard. I recognized it from a story I had read about Marie Krystoflak, who was inspired to engage with the gay community because of Mary, who, she believed, loved everyone, healthy or sick, gay or straight.

"We have a parish that is full of love and understanding," she said proudly in 1988. "We all belong to God."

When Marie died a decade later, the only request in her obituary was that friends send donations to the Most Holy Redeemer AIDS Support Group.

Inside the church, Father Donal Godfrey, a Jesuit priest with deep connections to the parish, gave me a tour of the sanctuary. By the entry was a table covered in old photographs, an All Souls' Day remembrance. My guide stopped and pointed at the photos of several gay men who had died from AIDS, some of them decades earlier. But each November, parishioners displayed the photos, intent on keeping the memories of their loved ones alive. We walked on to a side chapel filled with candles in the colors of a rainbow. A plaque pointed to an icon that Archbishop Quinn presented to the parish in 1995, the year AIDS deaths reached an all-time high in the United States. At that point, nearly 320,000 Americans had died from AIDS, which that year was the leading cause of death among people ages twenty-five to forty-four. The image shows Mary cradling the baby Jesus, who holds a candle in his hands. The icon is a copy of the one created by Father Bill McNichols, the same image that stands in Saint Francis Xavier back in New York. My journey to understand this part of the church's history had now taken me across an entire continent. And Father Bill McNichols's art accompanied me along the way.

There was one more item I wanted to see, so we left the side chapel and walked to a stained-glass window in the center of the sanctuary. Below it was a scroll with text written in deep red ink. The scroll lists the names of parishioners who had died from AIDS, young people who worshipped and grieved in this very space.

The scroll is prominently displayed, easily accessible by anyone who worships here today. It is clearly an important memento for the parish. I couldn't help but think of the hidden memorial I had seen back in New York, tucked away in a choir loft. This memorial offered such a contrast, flanked by a sizable bouquet of fresh yellow lilies and orange daisies. As I thought of the many gay men who had helped mold Most Holy Redeemer into a place that supported gay Catholics and their loved ones, I said a quiet prayer, thanking them for their struggle and wishing that more of them had survived to see the progress.

16

A CHURCH FILLED WITH GOSPEL LOVE

Something about Pope John Paul II spoke to Stephen Martz. He didn't seek out the Polish pope, but fate seemed to guide him to the steps of Saint Matthew's Cathedral in Washington, DC, on a Saturday morning in the fall of 1979. Inside the red brick church, the pope celebrated Mass in front of a crowd of 1,500 priests. More people, including Steve, stood outside, listening to the liturgy through speakers that had been set up to accommodate the overflow crowd, which included a group of gay and lesbian Catholics.

Steve hadn't been thinking much about religion in those days. Unlike the people who had lined up the night before to secure a spot that would allow a glimpse of the globe-trotting pope, Steve more or less stumbled upon the gathering. He was in his late twenties and on the staff of DC's gay newspaper, the *Blade*. He was comfortable with his sexual orientation, and he knew about the Catholic Church's hostility toward homosexuality. But that morning, after finishing his workout at the YMCA and finding himself near the cathedral, his mind drifted toward the spiritual. While listening to the pope and taking in the crowd's energy, he decided right then that he would become Catholic. The experience was as intense as it was unsettling. He seemed to be drowning in a rough sea of emotion. But he knew he had been called.

As luck would have it, Steve found a priest who ministered at the cathedral who happened also to identify as gay. The priest helped him understand the basics of Catholic theology and didn't scoff when Steve described what he felt were mystical experiences. Less than a year after that encounter with John Paul II, Steve was received into the Catholic Church. Then he dropped what felt like a bomb on his new friend.

"I think I'm being called to become a priest," he said.

Rather than dismiss Steve's call as the zeal of a convert, his friend encouraged him to explore opportunities to join a Catholic seminary. Steve was clear-eyed about the challenge that lay ahead. An editor of a gay newspaper was not exactly the ideal candidate for the Catholic priesthood. He was rejected by the Archdiocese of Washington, whose archbishop had been cracking down on gay and lesbian Catholics, but he kept looking, having learned that some religious orders tended to be more open to gay men. By 1984, the Claretians had accepted his application, and Steve packed up his desk at the *Blade* and moved to the Midwest to begin life as a novice.

That fall, Steve had to choose a ministry to undertake as part of the novitiate and he knew immediately that he was being called again, this time to HIV and AIDS care. By this point, he had heard the hurtful words from Catholic leaders about homosexuality. He knew the path he had chosen as an openly gay priest would not be easy, but he refused to hide his identity. And when he saw the gay community in need, he understood instinctively that he had to make life a bit easier for people suffering from AIDS. He told his religious community about his plans, and they were supportive.

For the next few months, Steve researched available resources for Chicagoans with HIV. He met with chaplains who were already engaged in AIDS ministry, often toiling on their own, including a gay priest who worked at a large hospital. He volunteered at the Howard Brown Memorial Clinic, which provided healthcare in the heart of Boystown. He was moved by the medical services he saw being offered to an underserved community but dismayed by the lack of pastoral resources available to patients. He understood that many gay men shed the religion of their youth when they came out publicly, often because institutional faith could be so homophobic. But he also suspected that facing a life-threatening illness without spiritual support could be hell.

"We identified very quickly that church institutions didn't really have credibility in the gay community," he remembers.

There was too much pain, he knew as well as anyone else. A close friend in Washington, who taught at the Catholic University of America, had been unable to reconcile his faith and his sexuality and turned to hooking up, often in unsafe ways, when the urge became too great. He eventually died from AIDS.

"The church's cruelty caused deaths of men who did not have to die," Steve recalled. The power of religion over some gay men could be extraordinary, and Steve vowed to do whatever he could to help heal those wounds.

A few dozen pastoral care providers, from a variety of faith traditions, gathered in Chicago in February of 1985 to talk about their experiences ministering to people with AIDS. A consensus quickly emerged.

"We needed a movement to make sure people with AIDS had access to good pastoral care regardless of what the church was doing," Steve remembers. Despite the harmful words against gay people coming from some church leaders, he knew that faith communities had to coordinate a pastoral response, because in Chicago, "the Catholic Church was a locus of both the positive and negative side of AIDS care."

Steve's mission was to tip the scales in the direction of the positive.

The group branded itself the AIDS Pastoral Care Network. Receiving financial support from Jewish and Protestant communities, plus several Catholic religious orders, its members met with patients and families in need of pastoral care, provided educational training about HIV and AIDS ministry, and lobbied for religious institutions to be more welcoming to gay people. When the Vatican released its anti-gay "Halloween letter" in 1986, Steve stood up for other gay Catholics, telling a *Chicago Tribune* reporter that he found the letter "disgusting" and warning that it would become "a powerful symbol of rejection" that might "transform gay people into modern-day lepers." He refused to mince words with so much on the line.

While enrolled in classes full-time, Steve spent the next few years helping the organization grow while also providing one-on-one support to people with AIDS who came from every segment of Chicago. It was John, a twenty-seven-year-old gay Jewish man, whose experience with AIDS most affected Steve.

John had been living in Texas but returned home to Chicago to die. By the time Steve met John, his face was covered in purple lesions. But he refused to let the unsightly marks limit him in what he knew would be his final weeks. They'd have dinner, maybe catch a movie downtown at the Chestnut Station Cinemas. As John's illness grew worse, Steve visited him at home, sitting on the floor next to his bed, the blinds closed tight because the light made everything hurt. They spent hours chatting, though sometimes John didn't have much energy, so Steve would stay in that dark apartment, quietly staring at a large poster taped to the wall. Advertising *Twelfth Night*, it depicted five gray trees set against a black backdrop, the roots of the trees writhing together, with a pale moon off in the sky. Steve stared at the image, zeroing in on the roots, meditating on the fact that AIDS had thrown so many random people together in these intense, personal relationships.

The morning John died, Steve received a call from John's brother giving him the news, and as his friend had previously requested, he headed over to the apartment to help take care of the arrangements. After John's body had been taken downstairs, Steve opened the blinds as the sun rose over Lake Michigan, natural light flooding the east-facing apartment. Steve had never seen the apartment so bright, and something caught his eye. A sunbeam fell directly on the poster.

"What I had never seen in all those nights and in all that darkness during the days he was dying, I now saw. Inside that moon, a lily," Steve recalled, reflecting on the flower's association with new life. "At that moment, I knew he was fine." Later, he would call that event "one of the most religious experiences of my life."

In some ways, Steve's short but intensely meaningful friendship with John was not unique. Other members of Chicago's AIDS Pastoral Care Network described similar encounters. They shared stories with one another, offering edification and support as the death toll mounted. But as a group, they knew the need for spiritual solace was greater than they could provide to individual clients. There was so much pain. The gay community, harmed by a seemingly limitless supply of religious bigotry, needed space to heal. That's when they turned to a Catholic parish not far from Boystown to host an event that they hoped would be a balm to Chicago's entire gay community.

———

It started as something of a publicity stunt: gay men into the leather subculture invading a Catholic church on Chicago's north side. The dynamic would raise eyebrows. But more importantly, it might bring some much-needed attention to the ongoing struggle against AIDS. Each Memorial Day weekend, thousands of gay men passionate about leather descended on Chicago for the International Mr. Leather (IML) contest and convention. Many of the participants were tired of feeling shunned by more mainstream gay rights groups. They understood why they were kept at arm's length, but they didn't like it.

The gay rights movement in the 1980s tried to show straight America that LGBT people really weren't so different. Gays and lesbians, the message went, wanted many of the same things as heterosexuals: an unencumbered right to love whomever they chose and freedom from workplace discrimination, access to healthcare, and the security of knowing they could not be evicted simply because they were gay.

The demands were reasonable, activists argued, just like gay and lesbian people.

One of the tactics to achieve these goals was assimilation. *We dress like you, we talk like you, we're already in your universities and your workplaces and your neighborhoods and your churches. You probably don't realize how many gay and lesbian people you already know.* There were obstacles in achieving those goals, of course, such as opposition from religious leaders, including Catholic bishops. But through the 1980s and '90s, progress finally felt within reach. Gay politics became respectable, and people seemed more open to so-called alternative lifestyles. Assimilation seemed to be working.

But not every segment of the gay community was on board with these tactics. Bulging with muscles and flaunting thick body hair, the leather community was about as in-your-face as it gets when it comes to sexuality. They skipped the polo shirts and khakis favored by more mainstream gays, opting instead for leather harnesses and tight denim. Their bars were dimly lit. Sex seemed to be everywhere.

International Mr. Leather was like any other convention in some ways—old friends caught up over cocktails and vendors displayed their latest wares. But there were key differences. Sex parties in hotel rooms. Condoms, porn, and leather goods for sale in the marketplace. And the main attraction of the weekend: a pageant crowning that year's International Mr. Leather.

In the 1980s, participants gathered inside a theatre for the main event, which could take hours, the auditorium hot and sweaty. A portion of the contest, like any other pageant, was dedicated to physical looks. Most of the Mr. Leather wannabees went shirtless, sporting black leather pants. Sometimes they wore even less. During speeches, judges and contestants bantered back and forth. Only twenty men would be selected as finalists and invited to the next round. It was like Miss America—but featuring muscly guys in tight pants and leather vests. The organization said the winner would be someone "who can best represent the community-at-large, the image of an openly gay man comfortable in his sexual orientation, for whom leathersex is a positive lifestyle." Or as Chicago's gay newspaper cheekily put it, the winner of International Mr. Leather would be "a hunk who can talk."

In the 1980s, more than half of Americans believed homosexual sex should be illegal and just a quarter said they knew a gay or lesbian friend, relative, or coworker. With their nipple clamps, provocative body piercings, and bare torsos, these gay men rejected this condemnation by embracing and even flaunting their sexuality.

In addition to the joy of knowing he was the object of desire of hundreds of men gathered in a Chicago hotel, the winner of International Mr. Leather also inherited various responsibilities that, beginning in the late 1980s, included attending an interfaith AIDS prayer service inside a Catholic church.

———

Starting in 1986, the AIDS Pastoral Care Network hosted a candlelight vigil each Memorial Day weekend. The service started at Saint Clement

Catholic Church and wound its way through Boystown. Though organizers understood the tension that existed between the gay community
and the Catholic Church, Saint Clement was large and centrally located.
Plus, the parish welcomed the group with open arms; it even had its own
AIDS ministry, with parishioners signing up to help run errands for the
homebound.

Chicago was hit by HIV and AIDS later than New York and San
Francisco, but the impact on its gay community became ferocious. In
Boystown, one person out of every three hundred was diagnosed with
HIV by the late 1980s. The candlelight procession effectively brought a
memorial service out into the streets. People would not be allowed to forget about those suffering silently. The vigil reminded people that suffering
was everywhere, even if the visible signs of sickness stayed mostly hidden
inside homes and clinics.

Leathermen knew something about making a scene. So when IML
organizers realized their event coincided with the vigil, they added one
more responsibility to the winner's portfolio. That year's Mr. Leather and
his fellow finalists would attend the church service and lead the candlelight procession. The city's mainstream gay activists would be present at
the vigil; now, so would the leather community. The leathermen were
intent on bringing visibility to their community's own struggle with
AIDS and demanding their place in the gay rights movement.

The IML finalists would need help traveling up to the church, and
Dean Ogren was perfect for the job, his two worlds suddenly colliding.
Like Steve Martz, Dean had converted to Catholicism as an adult, much
to the chagrin of his gay friends who pointed out that the Catholic Church
was not exactly friendly to leathermen. That didn't matter to Dean. He
relished being gay and he thrived in the leather world, fully embracing that
part of his life. When he became Catholic, he understood that the church
condemned his sexuality. But he was drawn to the church for other reasons.

"I like the pomp and circumstance of the Mass, the structure's organization, how the church talks about God," he said.

Dean reconciled his faith with his sexual orientation by ignoring condemnations of homosexuality from bishops and the Vatican. Many LGBT Catholics I've talked to have said the same thing. Some said they never heard anti-gay statements in their gay-friendly parishes, even back in the 1980s, so it never felt that difficult being gay and Catholic. As an adult convert to Catholicism, Dean said he could "kind of cherry pick" which aspects of the faith helped him foster a relationship with God. "I think that's how a lot of gay people have had to look at any religion, Catholic or otherwise," he said.

Back at IML weekend, Dean was unsure what lay in store for him and the leathermen he would accompany to the vigil, but he was eager to find out. He reminded the contestants that they had to be in good shape for church—limit the drugs and alcohol—and many took the responsibility seriously. Of course, the contestants had traveled to Chicago to party, see friends, and have sex. But all that was put on hold for a few hours. It was a small sacrifice given the seriousness of the epidemic. Many of the contestants had been raised in religious households themselves, and some of them still practiced, so they knew how to behave. Still, this wasn't just any ordinary religious service. The purpose was to remember the many gay men who had died from AIDS, a plague that struck the leather community especially hard.

The participants put on their Sunday best—though some embellished their outfits with a bit of leather flair—and made their way to the church. They decided that they wouldn't just melt into the crowd; they would be visible. Even if the more mainstream gay groups didn't want them in the front of their pride parades, even if leather bars were avoided by some gays who feared such overt and intense sexuality, the IML crowd would be seen here. At church.

Some priests and members of Dignity looked on in awe, and others with trepidation, as they watched the IML contestants enter the pews. Were they here to cause trouble? Was this a protest? What exactly was the message they wanted to deliver with their presence?

But as the men in leather took their seats, the service began. The mood was festive yet respectful. An African American Catholic children's choir waved brightly colored ribbons and raised their voices in song. A group of drummers provided a steady beat, reminding attendees that they must refuse to be silent in the face of AIDS.

It quickly became obvious that the leather crowd hadn't come to raise a ruckus. One priest in attendance marveled at their assertive but polite demeanor. He felt inspired that the crowd was comfortable being themselves, even in a Catholic church. "People shouldn't have to worry about being accepted for who they are," he thought to himself.

Chicago's gay community confronted its grief during the interfaith vigil. Clergy preached that AIDS was not a punishment from God, as some religious voices had alleged. The evening provided family and friends who had lost loved ones to AIDS an opportunity to gather together to weep, pray, and remember.

International Mr. Leather 1989, Guy Baldwin, remembers the vigils well. A therapist by trade, he had entered the contest more or less on a whim, thinking it might be a good platform to spread his call to political action. He had flown from his home in Los Angeles to Chicago. In his forties, Guy was among the oldest contestants, described as "a hunk for all seasons." Though other leathermen partied deep into the night, he was in bed by eleven. He had come to win the coveted IML title, and he wasn't taking any chances. He prevailed.

In speeches, he got political. He highlighted the need for honesty when it came to sexual expression and urged support for the pro-democracy movement in Eastern Europe, while reminding the leathermen not to let up in the fight against conservative politics here at home.

Even if Guy was angry at religious leaders for opposing gay rights and safer sex campaigns, he had a spiritual side. This became apparent during the service, when he was instructed to exit his pew and walk to one of three kneelers placed before ten-foot-tall banners, each with a drawing of a tree placed about halfway up. As the choir sang the hymn "Healer of Every Ill," those gathered inside Saint Clement's were invited to take a marker, kneel, and write below the trees the names of partners, loved ones, and friends they had lost to AIDS, the names blending together to form strong roots.

Guy certainly hadn't been prepared to confront the pain of losing hundreds of lovers, friends, clients, and acquaintances. That grief seemed at times unbearable, and he had learned to push down those feelings whenever he could, letting his emotions flow out back in the safety of his home.

But now, inside this church, in a very public setting, he made his way to the kneelers, selecting the one on the far left. He grabbed a marker and began writing. His whole mind went into the task, the service around him dissolving into a blur. He thought of the partner he had lost. He recalled the clients who had asked him to visit them in the hospital, where he had placed his leather coat on their beds before carrying out their wishes to be removed from ventilators. He remembered stopping at the grocery store right after one of those traumatizing experiences and looking aghast as people put boxes of cereal and bottles of juice into their carts, oblivious to the plague taking place all around them.

Back in the church, he felt traumatized, like someone had shoved his hands into a burning pile of coals. He thought of all the people whose names he had just written, of all the inaction that caused so much suffering and death, and he was angry. Now, it was time to transform that anger into action, to end the willful ignorance that infected so much of society.

As the service ended, congregants carried lit candles and placed them below the banners inscribed with the names of those who had died from

AIDS. The lights dimmed. The flickering flames threw shadows throughout the church.

Leading the procession through the neighborhood was that year's International Mr. Leather. He sported leather gear and his sash and medallions, signs that he had triumphed over all the other contestants to claim his title. He held a candle and dozens of leathermen followed. Some held hands, others kissed. Priests and nuns walked behind. It was a scene of quiet reverence for lost lives, led by determined people who refused to let society sweep their suffering under the rug.

————

In a report written for Cardinal Joseph Bernardin in 1986, Steve Martz and his colleagues on the archdiocese's AIDS Task Force, including Father Jim Noone, soberly reported, "AIDS has hit the gay community even more sharply in Chicago than in most cities," citing the higher proportion of gay men comprising the city's HIV cases compared to the national average. The report also notes that many people with AIDS had been victimized by "fundamentalist" theology that cruelly told them that "AIDS is God's punishment."

For Steve, this was a sin.

Before joining his religious order, he had been an editor at a gay newspaper. He knew well the tensions that existed between the gay community and religious institutions, but he believed that both could benefit from each other. Early on, when he tried volunteering at a local clinic serving primarily gay men, the staff had been skeptical of his motivations. They wanted to keep faith leaders far away from their clients. As Steve observed, while gay people were no longer considered criminals or mentally ill as they had been just decades earlier, most religious bodies still considered them sinners. He understood the skepticism.

But he also knew many gay people who still desired the support of a faith community. Sadly, many had felt "that to come out of the closet one had to put God in that closet." And at a time when so many young gay people would have benefitted from spiritual sustenance during their final days, Steve was insistent that religious leaders do better. As he pressed publicly for greater acceptance, he also connected with other Catholic leaders so that together they could provide spiritual care and support for a community in need, whether at packed Memorial Day vigils or during quieter moments in lakefront high-rises. The response was never perfect, and Steve would eventually leave his Catholic religious order and go on to become an Episcopal priest.

But as he described it to me years later, "As ugly and as horrible and as painful as those years were, in part because too many Church leaders would not see Christ in their dying gay brothers, and even with the many tears that were shed, there was another Catholic Church, closer to the cross, whose response was loving and compassionate and beautiful, full of gospel love."

17

"JUST WHO THE HELL ARE THESE TWO NUNS?"

When Sister Carol and Sister Mary Ellen returned home to Belleville, Illinois, they put to work the lessons learned at Saint Vincent's and Saint Clare's, on the hotline, and through conversations with their new friends who had introduced them to New York gay life, Will and Jim. They reviewed their notes from their stays in Kansas City and Chicago and then decided to open a drop-in center, a place where people with HIV and AIDS could visit, knowing they would not be judged. There, guests could meet with a nurse, ask questions of a social worker, or maybe just relax. When the hospital run by their religious order offered them an empty office building across the street, Sister Carol and Sister Mary Ellen jumped at the opportunity. That would take care of a potentially costly and time-consuming real estate hunt. As they checked each item off their to-do list, they were confident that they were ready to assist Belleville in responding to what they anticipated would be a growing need for HIV and AIDS care.

On an otherwise quiet day following the opening of the new center, Sister Carol heard a soft knocking at the back door. She walked down the hallway and looked outside, where she saw a man standing, sinking into his trench coat and pulling his hat down tightly over his head. The building was located on a busy street, the front door in clear view of the passing cars and nearby pedestrians. He knew he needed help, and he had already driven by a few times, but he had been too nervous to stop. He had felt too exposed with so many eyes around. But today was the day, he told himself. He was going to go inside. Still, there was no way he would use the front door, so he walked to the rear of the building, seeking the counsel of a Catholic nun who, he had heard, would help people like him, people who had just been diagnosed with HIV and had nowhere else to turn.

"Hi, I'm Sister Carol. How can I help you?"

She listened to the man's story. He was scared. Doctors refused to see him.

"I can help with that."

The man didn't know how to process his feelings about his HIV diagnosis.

"I know other people in the same situation," Sister Carol reassured him, sounding newly confident in her ability to help. "Maybe you can all meet?"

The man felt safer after a few minutes talking to Sister Carol. He finally opened up a bit and told her his name.

"I'm John, by the way."

John explained that entering through a front door on a busy street was too much to ask of people who were beaten down by the stigma associated with HIV. Sister Carol made a mental note, a consequence of small-town life she and Mary Ellen had failed to take into account as they planned their opening.

It turned out that John wasn't the only person who was unwilling to make use of that front door. Letter carriers refused to carry in mail.

Other clients didn't want to be seen visiting. Even some otherwise well-meaning medical professionals asked for a more discreet location to discuss client needs. Sister Carol realized that despite the intense six months in New York, she and Sister Mary Ellen still needed more help if they were to become effective allies in Belleville's still-nascent fight against HIV. AIDS ministry in New York had been one thing. Back here in Belleville, it was something else entirely.

Savvy enough to understand that their ministry would benefit from the blessing of the diocese, they kept the local bishop in the loop. They had previously filled him in about their plans before they left for New York and updated him once they returned. Before they opened their drop-in center, they asked for financial support, which they received. (The one hiccup came when Sister Carol, who always spoke her mind, told the bishop that she had met some priests in New York who were HIV-positive. She asked him, "Do you know what your gay priests are up to?" He retorted, "I wouldn't have the faintest idea and I'd be the last to know." Carol immediately understood that AIDS and the priesthood was not yet a topic that Catholics in Belleville were ready to confront.)

When it came to naming the new center, Sister Carol turned to her faith, reflecting on what she understood as her Christian duty to respond compassionately to people with AIDS. One place mentioned repeatedly in the gospels stuck with Sister Carol and Sister Mary Ellen: the village of Bethany.

The nuns believed that Bethany, situated just over the Mount of Olives from Jerusalem, was akin to a leper colony. Jesus dines at the house of "Simon the Leper" while staying in Bethany, and in the 1980s, the two nuns saw the mistreatment of people with AIDS through this lens. Bethany was also where Jesus had raised his friend Lazarus from the dead and where he was anointed before his crucifixion. All this suggested that Bethany was the perfect inspiration for the new center.

As Carol put it, Bethany was where "Jesus came to be with his friends, to kick off his sandals, put up his feet, have a beer."

That was the atmosphere they were going for, somewhere that people with AIDS could be with friends, insulated from shame and stigma, and perhaps forget momentarily about their trials. They decided to call the new center Bethany Place.

Ahead of their opening, Sister Carol and Sister Mary Ellen transformed the empty rooms into a reception area to make it as comfortable as possible. In a small office space, they set up an AIDS hotline modeled on the GMHC version in New York. They met with the health department to make sure they had the most up-to-date information about HIV testing. They visited sites to see which ones were most professional before they referred future clients. They talked to doctors and nurses, intent on being good partners in the fight against AIDS.

On Bethany Place's first day, a skinny guy with a boom box resting on his shoulder walked in.

"I'm Anthony, and I have AIDS."

"Well hi, Anthony, come on in."

Anthony told Sister Carol and Sister Mary Ellen that he was having trouble finding a doctor, because many refused to take on patients with AIDS. The excuses they offered varied. Some of it was discrimination, some of it was fear, and some just didn't want to scare off their other patients. The nuns thought of a friend at one of the larger local hospitals who treated people with AIDS. They called and asked if she'd be willing to see Anthony. She said yes.

Bethany Place had successfully served its first client. Maybe this wouldn't be so difficult after all. In many ways, the experience made sense. Sister Carol and Sister Mary Ellen had sought out local resources, then moved to New York for more insight. When they arrived back home, they connected with all the healthcare agencies, hospitals, and doctors they could find. Then they opened their doors and waited for clients. In walked Anthony, and the two nuns found him a doctor.

Sister Carol kept at it. She worked the phones, trying to find additional doctors to care for her clients. She fought with nursing homes to accept patients with AIDS when they needed round-the-clock care. She badgered lawyers to visit hospital rooms to draw up wills. All that work created an aura of tenacity around Carol. Sure, she could talk sweetly about the gospel and Saint Francis, but when her clients needed assistance, she was relentless. She tracked down people in power and asked them to help her clients repeatedly until they gave in. Some doctors and administrators who would rather not work with people with AIDS referred to her derisively behind her back as "*that* woman."

Sister Carol and Sister Mary Ellen's early clients were pleased with the assistance, but there still just weren't that many people visiting Bethany Place. The nuns had done their research before they opened. There were definitely more people in Belleville living with HIV who could use their help. So where were they?

———

Despite all their planning, Sister Carol and Sister Mary Ellen had failed to reach one core constituency who might be well served by Bethany Place. The two nuns simply didn't know many gay men. And at this point, in 1988, gay men made up the vast majority of new HIV and AIDS diagnoses. It was not necessarily a community innately inclined to trust a pair of Catholic nuns. That began to change with a single phone call from someone in desperate need.

The caller, who refused to give his name, planned to drive five hours from Belleville to Chicago, because he was too afraid to seek AIDS care near his home. He only made it about ten miles before he felt too sick to continue. He had been given Sister Carol's name as someone who could help. Yes, she was a Catholic nun, but she wouldn't ask any questions about why he was sick.

"I'm HIV-positive," he disclosed, "and I need to see a doctor." He explained that he was from a prominent family in town, and no one could know he was sick.

And there was one more thing he wanted to tell Sister Carol: "I'm not gay!"

Sister Carol ignored that last comment. Her time in New York had taught her to avoid any kind of language that could convey judgment and possibly alienate someone in need of medical help.

"Well, first of all, you've got to get yourself back here," she said. "I'll arrange to get you admitted to Saint Elizabeth's immediately."

Sister Carol found a bed for the man, who told her his name was Christopher, at Saint Elizabeth's. Over the course of their visits, which became daily as he grew sicker, they developed a friendship. Christopher saw that Sister Carol was compassionate, working hard to find care for a complete stranger. She was also trustworthy and willing to be discreet. Because of those visits, Christopher felt comfortable introducing Sister Carol to his friend George, a bartender at one of Belleville's gay bars, Lil's. The three of them became fast friends.

"You've got to come down to the bar one night," the two men told Sister Carol.

Sister Carol had visited gay bars in Chelsea and Hell's Kitchen. Surely she could handle Belleville's. She took Christopher and George up on their offer. If she wanted to help the gay community in Belleville, she understood that she had to meet them first on their turf.

For their part, Christopher and George wanted their friends to know they had a trusted ally in Sister Carol. One way to show their trust, while also helping her fledgling ministry, was to host a fundraiser at the bar. But when word got out about the event, some of the gays in Belleville were not pleased.

"Just who the hell are these two nuns?" they demanded.

"Trust us," Christopher and George begged their friends. But it would take more time to win them over.

One afternoon while Sister Carol was in her office, a thin man, more than six-and-a-half-feet tall, stormed in. He slammed the door behind him.

"I want to talk to you," he snarled. "I want to know where this money is going. The Catholic Church is taking it, isn't it?"

Sister Carol stared in disbelief. Who was this guy? And what was he talking about?

"Well, hello. Who are you?"

"I'm Ted."

"Hi, Ted."

He explained that he lived across the river in St. Louis and that he worked at a hair salon. He had heard that Christopher and George were organizing a "cut-a-thon," with the proceeds from haircuts supporting a new AIDS center run by a couple of nuns.

"The church is stealing money from the gay community!"

Sister Carol suddenly understood.

"The hospital manages our books," she patiently explained. State grants paid for half her salary, and the other half, well, she simply volunteered. She offered to show Ted their financial records so he could see for himself that any donated money didn't go to the diocese. Plus, she said she understood the bigotry that could be present in town. Many times, when people found out she worked in HIV and AIDS care, they'd ask her why, their voices tinged with suspicion. Some were more direct and simply accused her of being gay. Sister Carol brushed it off. "That's for me to know and you to find out. That has nothing to do with what we're dealing with here."

By the end of the conversation, Ted seemed convinced that Sister Carol and Sister Mary Ellen knew what they were doing, and more importantly, that they were on the side of the gay and lesbian community. That seemed to be enough for Ted. He said he was on board with Bethany Place and asked how he could help.

The outreach to the gay community seemed to work, as soon enough, the number of clients seeking help from Bethany Place increased. As Sister Carol rightly predicted, even Belleville, nestled away in southern Illinois, wasn't immune to the ongoing crisis. The nuns soon realized they could fill a need by offering more robust public education about HIV and AIDS.

Overwhelming fear of the epidemic seemed rampant in Belleville, much of it based on a misunderstanding of how the virus spread. An early client at Bethany Place was a thirty-nine-year-old man who contracted HIV while living in California. He had moved home to southern Illinois when he developed AIDS and turned to Bethany Place for assistance. He was hospitalized, but he left one afternoon to visit his family at an outdoor picnic. Later in the day, back in the office, the phone rang. A woman told Sister Mary Ellen through sobs that she was the man's stepmother. She said that at the end of the picnic, the family dog had scarfed down her stepson's leftover food.

"Could the dog get AIDS?" she asked.

Sister Mary Ellen couldn't believe what she was hearing. If she and Sister Carol had harbored any residual doubts about the great need for HIV education in Belleville, they were now gone.

They decided to host workshops at Bethany Place. They wanted to give people at risk of contracting HIV information about how best to protect themselves and for those who wanted to volunteer, they provided insight that they had picked up during their visits to GMHC in New York. And for the wider community, their message was simple: don't panic.

Sister Carol patiently explained how HIV was spread, not shying away from words no one expected to come from a short, Polish nun: semen, anal sex, condoms. Her audiences often fidgeted uncomfortably, especially the high schoolers. But Sister Carol feared the students were at high risk because nobody would tell them the truth about AIDS. She knew they had to understand the science about the disease if the fear and stigma were to go away anytime soon. And to that end, Sister Carol always started her talks with one rule, something she had learned in New York.

"Before you can effectively minister to anyone with HIV or AIDS," she explained, "you need to look at your own biases and make sure you're seeing the person in front of you, not their disease or how they contracted HIV."

That was a lesson Belleville had not yet fully embraced.

———

Anthony, the first client who had walked through the door at Bethany Place with his boom box, returned again and again over the next several months. Sister Carol had taken a liking to Anthony, so when he called one day to say he didn't feel well—that he had been growing weaker in recent weeks—she asked if he could get himself to the hospital.

"I don't think I can make it on my own," he said.

"I'll be right there," Carol told him.

A priest volunteering at Bethany Place joined Sister Carol for the drive, which took them into East St. Louis, where Anthony lived in a neighborhood with high rates of poverty and crime. When they arrived at Anthony's house, they found that the windows and doors were covered in bars. Sister Carol knocked. No answer. They knocked louder, then tried to open the door themselves. The bars were dead-bolted shut.

Finally, a gaunt figure made his way to the door, using what looked like an ancient castle key to open the gate.

"Oh my God, Anthony," Carol said, her voice mixed with both fright and relief. "You're going to die in this house, and no one would be able to get in to help."

"I know, I know. But see those guys? They know I'm gay and that I have AIDS. They hang out over there 'cause they want to kick the crap out of me."

"Well, get in the car, we're taking you to the hospital."

A couple of days later, Sister Carol and another sister who ministered at Bethany Place drove to the hospital to visit Anthony.

When they arrived, they were horrified by what they encountered. The room stank of human waste and the bedsheets hadn't been cleaned in, based on the smell, many days. The hospital staff was clearly neglecting Anthony. He looked even sicker than when Sister Carol had picked him up at home a couple of days earlier. He deserved better than this. The nuns, both nurses by training, jumped into action. They cleaned Anthony, found fresh bedding, and did what they could to make the room sparkle.

In walked a minister. He was there to visit Anthony, apparently, but Sister Carol didn't recognize him.

"Did you guys pray with him yet?" he asked the two nuns.

It took everything Sister Carol had not to scream.

"Pray? We've been cleaning him up because people are too afraid to touch him because he has AIDS."

The minister shrugged his shoulders.

"Well, I'm here to pray."

Sister Carol took a deep breath. She was still a nun, after all. While she was furious at the state of Anthony's room—and now at this minister who had visited previously but left him to sit in his own waste—she believed prayer was important.

"OK, we'll pray."

The three of them, two Catholic nuns and a Pentecostal minister, held hands and stood around Anthony's now clean bed. They prayed for him. Later that night, Anthony, the first client to walk through the doors of Bethany Place, who had helped Sister Carol understand the needs of gay men dying from AIDS, took his last breath.

Sister Carol was saddened by Anthony's death, but it became clear his would be but one of a seemingly endless string of lives cut short around Belleville. By this point, there were many clients in need of her attention and dozens of volunteers waiting to undergo training. The fundraising was going well, with regular walk-a-thons and candlelight vigils, Christmas parties, and social events. At the same time, Carol felt like funerals were filling up her calendar. She tried to attend them all—including, eventually, a funeral for an early advocate of Bethany Place who had become one of Sister Carol's good friends.

———

Sister Carol was chatting with Christopher and George one Friday afternoon when Christopher suddenly collapsed, falling right to the floor. When he came to after a second, Sister Carol could tell he was embarrassed.

"Christopher, I knew you liked me, but now you've really fallen for me," she said.

The silly joke made him smile, but it was clear that he was really sick. He had been diagnosed with HIV a couple years earlier, and now he had developed AIDS.

Christopher's life was representative of the complexity of gay life in places like Belleville. Though George was his boyfriend, he also had a wife and two children and did not disclose to many people that he was bisexual. Knowing the end was now near, he wanted to be honest with them about his struggle. By this point, he had moved in with George. He explained to his two sons, not yet teenagers, that he was sick and that he was dying. The news devastated his family. But during the next few months, Christopher's children spent the weekends with him and George, getting to know their father in a different light and affirming their dad's decision to be honest with his family.

With the end near, Christopher again turned to Sister Carol. Though raised Catholic, he wasn't a regular churchgoer. During his illness, he had relied on Sister Carol for spiritual support, even if it was less formal than worshipping in a church. But now, he wanted more.

"I'll help find you a priest," Sister Carol told her dying friend.

When Christopher passed away, at just thirty-seven, Sister Carol accompanied George to pick out a casket and helped him decide which mismatched socks Christopher would wear at his burial, a final homage to one of his silly sartorial flourishes. She worked with the parish to make sure Christopher would receive a proper Catholic funeral. She helped plan the memorial service that preceded the Mass. And as a final gift, Sister Carol took her flute and played a funereal send-off, a version of "The Rose," a song Christopher had loved during the final years of his life.

Though Sister Carol was a talented nurse, her AIDS ministry was never really about medicine. Nor was her mission shuffling paperwork, though she helped lots of young gay men find doctors and dentists. Sister Carol's ministry was about helping a young gay man come out to his mother before he died. Or calling to check in on another client a few times each week, and when he said he missed belting out Whitney Houston at karaoke, driving him to a gay bar so he could feel like his old self one more time. It was about assuring the many gay men who felt shame and stigma that she was on their side. Sister Carol's ministry was about love.

———

Sister Carol stayed on at Bethany Place for several years, watching with sadness as HIV spread through Belleville, just as she and Sister Mary Ellen had warned, affecting first the gay community and later IV drug users. By 1991, the surrounding area was home to the highest number of AIDS cases in Illinois outside of metropolitan Chicago. Women and children were regular clients. Some of the volunteers who had been trained at Bethany Place became activists themselves, evidence of the success of Sister Carol's and Sister Mary Ellen's educational outreach. Sister Carol felt she had found her calling, putting her nursing know-how, pastoral instinct, and knack for getting what she wanted to work for the good of a marginalized community.

Yet Bethany Place seemed to lurch from one financial crisis to another. There were unanticipated costs of running the AIDS ministry. Then when grants looked like they would be the answer, reams of paperwork overtook Sister Carol's schedule. By 1994, when it became clear that professional managers were needed to help Bethany Place find more solid footing, she stepped away.

———

By the time I met Carol in 2016, she had left her religious order. Through all our interviews and phone calls and emails, I could never quite get her to open up about why she had done this. She said the split felt like "a painful divorce," and she chose to leave it at that. Today she lives on her own and belongs to the Sisters for Christian Community, an international network that attracts many women who have left traditional religious life. Though she left her order, she still has contact with some of the sisters, including Sister Thomas Kundmueller, who had accompanied her to Anthony's hospital room decades earlier. When I ask if she still considers herself Catholic, she doesn't pause. "Oh yeah, I'll live and die a Catholic."

During a visit to Belleville, Carol took me to see Bethany Place, which is still in operation, though in a different location as its mission has evolved to meet new needs. It's housed in a "Quonset hut," a corrugated semicylindrical building, though the inside is comfortable. Clients hang out on oversized couches, relaxing music plays softly, and a light lavender scent fills the air. Like many AIDS organizations started by Catholics in the 1980s, Bethany Place is now independent, no longer affiliated with any religious order. But Sister Thomas still volunteers there, and a sense of Franciscan devotion appears to animate the mission.

Bethany Place's continued existence long after Carol departed is a stark reminder that HIV and AIDS are not consigned to the past. The center was able to help clients for so long because of Carol's journey decades ago. Back in the 1980s, Sister Carol didn't have to respond to AIDS. She could have ignored the crisis altogether or maybe learned the bare minimum to keep her boss at the home nursing agency satisfied. Perhaps she could have done what some other doctors and nurses did back then and requested not to treat people with AIDS at all.

But she didn't. Sister Carol listened to people in need, and she went out of her way to help. More than three decades later, Bethany Place still served its community. And though Carol is no longer a Catholic sister in the traditional sense, and though her health is in decline, she still ministers, this time to another young gay man seeking spiritual insight.

18

AIDS CRUCIFIXION

Father Bill McNichols moved to New York in 1980 to be an artist. In some ways, his years-long commitment to HIV and AIDS ministry put those plans on hold. After all, many days he woke up before dawn to visit patients in their homes before heading to the hospital, then met a friend with AIDS later in the day for dinner, and maybe squeezed in another visit or two before bed. On top of that ministry, Father Bill was a chaplain for Dignity, and later, he held healing Masses. Though he was young and energetic, there were only so many hours in the day, and AIDS ministry was emotionally draining work. That didn't leave much time for art. Or, at least, that was the impression Father Bill gave me in our early conversations.

But I questioned this assumption after reading a book by the Jesuit peace activist Daniel Berrigan. Father Berrigan had befriended Bill while they both lived in New York in the 1980s. Father Bill talked about his AIDS ministry with Berrigan during a ride on the subway, Bill's soft voice barely rising above the squealing brakes and rumble of wheels. But

Dan, as Bill called him in recounting the story, was hooked. He had protested the Vietnam War and led demonstrations against nuclear weapons. Berrigan, nearly three decades older than Bill, now wanted to minister to people with AIDS and sought advice from his younger Jesuit brother.

Berrigan went on to chronicle in his books his friendships with young gay men dying from AIDS. He found the experiences both moving and painful. He also wrote that he learned about the need for compassion toward people with AIDS through Father Bill's art. In his autobiography, Berrigan described how his friends with AIDS found comfort in Father Bill's drawings, which, he wrote, "shed light in dark corners—where, because of the present atmosphere of panic, many prefer to cower." Maybe Father Bill, in his "nervous, darting way," as Berrigan described him in his book, was being too self-effacing with me when I asked how his art helped people.

Father Bill had mailed me another box of materials, including old newspaper clippings, a dated issue of *Time* magazine, and notes he had jotted down over the years. I thumbed through everything, and I was struck by a slightly yellowed piece of cardboard the size of a sheet of printer paper. Taped in the middle is a drawing of Our Lady of Guadalupe, with a beautiful, handwritten script surrounding the frame.

It took a little research to figure out what I was holding, but I soon realized it was the master copy of the flyer advertising Father Bill's healing Masses from 1987. In that moment, I felt as if I held in my hands a holy relic. The past had come alive through conversations with people like Father Bill, Sister Carol, and David Pais. Contemporaneous newspaper accounts provided color, preserving small details that had slipped the minds of the people I interviewed—the names of hymns sung at a funeral or anecdotes about protesters bundling up to stave off the cold. But there was something about holding a piece of this history that transported me to a time I had been too young to remember firsthand.

How many people with AIDS and their loved ones had seen this exact flyer, the one now sitting on a shelf in my condo in Chicago? The flyer's very existence brought them to a church for comfort and healing. Decades later, by running my fingertips over this piece of cardboard, I felt a similar sensation that came from sitting in the room that had hosted the AIDS support group at Most Holy Redeemer and walking the grounds at the former Saint Vincent's Hospital. That's when it occurred to me that Father Bill's art had not gone dormant at all during the AIDS crisis; it just took on a different form. What I now held was, in some ways, just a flyer. Yellowed, worth no money. But to me, it served as a powerful example of how Father Bill's creativity helped alleviate fear around HIV, connecting the struggle of those suffering from AIDS with powerful religious imagery. That helped move people to compassion, ideally, by prompting them to consider the call to love their neighbor—especially their neighbors suffering with AIDS.

What is perhaps Father Bill's most famous image from that period is a drawing of the Blessed Virgin Mary, created in the style of traditional Eastern iconography. She wears a crimson robe, looking down at the child Jesus, draped in white and sitting on her lap. Golden halos surround each of their heads. Jesus stares out, locking eyes with you as you gaze on the icon. In many ways, it is a traditional and perhaps even unremarkable representation of Mary and Jesus, a pairing that has been created by many artists countless times over the centuries. But there is one small detail in Father Bill's image that sets it apart, a flourish that makes the icon meaningful to Catholics affected by HIV and AIDS. I saw copies of this icon in New York at Saint Francis Xavier, and then again in San Francisco at Most Holy Redeemer, and even here in Chicago at a parish in Boystown.

Jesus holds in his small hands a single candle, its flame golden yellow. Upon closer inspection, it is the same candle that Father Bill created for a flyer advertising an AIDS vigil years earlier. Father Bill called the icon *Mother of God, Light in All Darkness.* Those suffering from the physical reality of HIV and AIDS, in addition to the stigma associated with the disease, were promised in this icon the glowing light of God's love. Love that we here on earth are called to provide.

Father Bill had continued to create art during the HIV and AIDS crisis. That much was now clear to me. But I still wanted to hear from people who had been moved by his creativity at the height of the epidemic.

———

On a Friday night in April 1988, about 120 people gathered on the campus of Fordham University in New York. Students took a break from their usual boisterous weekend activities for something more somber: a Mass and candlelight vigil for people. A graduate student had suggested that campus ministry host the vigil, as he wanted Fordham to do more to remember and support those with HIV and AIDS.

The vigil began on Friday evening with an opening Mass celebrated by the school's president. At no time were fewer than twenty people holding vigil. Some participants read aloud the first names of people struggling with their HIV and AIDS diagnoses. At another point, the students participated in a traditional Catholic ritual called the Stations of the Cross, albeit a version that was designed precisely for this kind of moment.

The Stations of the Cross are a series of fourteen images recalling the passion and death of Jesus. Often, the stations are observed during Lent, when devotees pray with them by reflecting on the events depicted in each image. A selection of Scripture and a prayer commemorate each scene before congregants move on to the next station.

During the AIDS vigil at Fordham, those gathered to pray the stations used this centuries-old form of prayer to seek help in understanding the epidemic. Each of the fourteen moments was depicted in the form of someone suffering from AIDS. The reflections and prayers highlighted the personal struggles accompanying a new HIV diagnosis, becoming sick from AIDS, and ultimately dying from complications related to the disease. The creator of this unusual Stations of the Cross was a young Jesuit priest working on the AIDS ward at Saint Vincent's Hospital, Father Bill McNichols.

A controversial Catholic leader who had supported the gay and lesbian community, Archbishop Raymond G. Hunthausen of Seattle, wrote the foreword to the text. Partly because of his support for LGBT Catholics, Hunthausen had been subjected to a Vatican investigation in 1983 and then stripped of some authority. He was not silenced by that pressure, however, and continued to lend his support to efforts that embraced gay Catholics. Archbishop Hunthausen's endorsement of Father Bill's *The Stations of the Cross of a Person with AIDS* also signaled support from a senior church leader to Catholics who might face opposition in their efforts to minister to the gay and lesbian community.

In Father Bill's stations, the reflections center around Robert, a composite character Father Bill created. The images are simple, red ink on beige paper. In the traditional first station of the fourteen, Jesus is condemned to death. In Father Bill's version, Robert goes to the doctor to find out why he is experiencing frightening symptoms. He, too, learns that he is going to die.

Each successive moment of Jesus's life follows this pattern. Jesus carries his cross; Robert's mind races when he realizes he will confront his illness on his own. Jesus falls for the first time; Robert goes to an empty apartment, feeling like he has no one to help him, and drinks himself to sleep. Simon helps Jesus carry his cross; Robert attends a GMHC meeting and gets connected to a counselor. Women weep over Jesus; a kindly Catholic sister attends to Robert in the hospital. Jesus is stripped of his garments; Robert begins treatment for Kaposi's sarcoma. Jesus is nailed to the cross; Robert's cancer progresses, and he calls a priest to help plan his funeral. Jesus, rejected by society, dies; Robert experiences a vision of healing and comfort. Jesus's lifeless body is placed in his mother's arms; Robert, gravely ill, refuses to be connected to a ventilator and dies in his mother's arms. Jesus rises from the dead; Robert is one of many thousands of people whose memories live on.

———

Father Bill's AIDS-inspired art moved well beyond Fordham's campus and New York City into the many other places where gay men, and later people addicted to drugs, fought for their lives. In 1987, Stephen McDonnell tested positive for HIV. He was a twenty-nine-year-old gay man in Toronto who was racked with nerves about his health but too terrified to tell many people in his life. He had seen the way others talked about people with AIDS—not just the religiously motivated bigots he encountered, but even other gay men. He didn't want to face the exclusion he imagined in his future should people find out he was living with HIV. He prayed for death, hoping pneumonia would take him quickly, hoping to avoid the physical suffering and loneliness he witnessed in friends who had already died.

Like many gay Catholics, Stephen struggled to reconcile his faith with his sexual orientation. He knew about the church's letter condemning homosexuality and had heard the horror stories of dying gay men being condemned by heartless clerics. But still, there was something about his Catholic faith that captivated him, that made him want to figure out how to make life as a gay believer work. Stephen's search led him to a group of gay and bisexual Catholic men who met for prayer and socializing. It was here that Stephen began to feel less like an orphan, finding a community of people who understood his journey. Murmurings clued him in that a few others were also HIV-positive, but even among his peers, who celebrated gay life, revealing one's positive status felt taboo. Stigma from the outside had been internalized and the resulting shame was too powerful.

Many gay Catholics in the 1980s hunted down copies of *The Church and the Homosexual*, a book written in 1976 by the controversial Jesuit priest

Father John J. McNeill. In it, Father McNeill argued that the church should be more welcoming to its gay members because homophobia was rooted in an errant understanding of the Bible. Members of Stephen's prayer group devoured the book. They wanted to meet this prophet and hear more. They pooled their money and brought him to Toronto to lead a retreat.

During the retreat, Stephen was asked to imagine how Jesus would respond to gay and lesbian Catholics. This was not easy for him, as his conceptions of God had been shaped by a church hostile to people like him. But he took a deep breath and kept listening. Surely God would speak to him when the time was right. At one point, Father McNeill passed around copies of a pamphlet. It was a version of the Stations of the Cross that Stephen had never before seen, pen and ink drawings with accompanying text.

A few words leapt out right away to Stephen: gay, AIDS, love. Positive representations of gay people were so rare in the church. Yet Father Bill McNichols's gay-friendly Stations of the Cross, presented by a priest who said gay people were worthy of love, offered a message that was simple yet revolutionary: people with HIV and AIDS must not be shunned, but embraced. Stephen looked at the images that accompanied the stations. He sat for a moment taking this all in, realizing he was on the verge of something powerful. That's when another drawing in the pamphlet caught his eye.

At first glance, it was a simple black-and-white rendering of a crucifix, an image a Catholic like Stephen would have seen countless times in churches. But something about this particular drawing caught his attention. A cartoon sun and moon with despondent faces hurtle toward Jesus, who hangs lifeless on the cross. He is depicted speaking the words made known in Scripture, "Father, forgive them, they know not what they do" (Luke 23:34). There are figures on either side of the cross. Mary holds a sick man on one side, her shawl covered in stars. The ailing man is dressed in modern, almost trendy, attire. On the other side, a man wears a suit, his face twisted in rage. He shoves a book up toward the crucified Jesus. If you squint, it's clear that it's the Bible.

The crown of thorns is there, and Jesus's head hangs lifelessly to the side, but something is different about this Jesus: his near-naked body is covered in dark bruises. At the retreat, Stephen recognized them instantly as KS lesions. This Christ was unlike anything Stephen had ever seen. This Christ had AIDS. Above him, a sign revealed why he was being left to suffer and die: AIDS. HOMOSEXUAL. FAGGOT. PERVERT. SODOMITE.

Stephen snapped out of his daze as the group prayed through the stations. As they read aloud the life of Robert, from diagnosis to death, Stephen thought about his own journey. He struggled to keep his emotions in check during the prayer, not wanting to draw attention. For the first time in his life, Stephen saw images that allowed him to reconcile the love of his faith instilled in him as a young boy with the gay man he had become. Through those images, he told me, he felt God saying to him, "Stephen, I see you. I understand who you are. I accept you. I love you. And I will be with you on your journey."

He could have fallen to the ground. He just had to make it through the end of the retreat. He wasn't ready to explain to the group why he found the images and the prayers so powerful, that they spoke to him so personally. But that night, he took out the pamphlet, looked at the images one more time, and re-read the prayers. Then, alone in his room, finally able to release his pent-up emotion, Stephen wept.

———

Father Bill McNichols created many images related to HIV and AIDS during the roughly seven years he lived and worked in New York. In addition to *AIDS Crucifixion*, there is *The Epiphany: Wisemen Bring Gifts to the Child*. At the center of the drawing is the Virgin of Guadalupe, a nod to the church where Father Bill held his healing Masses. Draped in stars and ensconced by a rainbow, she holds the baby Jesus, who reaches out to someone who is too weak to sit up, assisted by Saint Francis of Assisi. The figure is based on a gay man with AIDS Father Bill met early in his ministry. On the other side of Mary stands Saint Aloysius, the Jesuit saint whose statue Father Bill kept in his office, holding a body covered in purple lesions. That man is based on a person Bill knew who contracted HIV through IV drug use. Images of hope and resurrection, including Easter lilies, the rainbow, and some wishbones, fill the scene. Bill said the image was "aimed like an arrow to elicit compassion, about people with AIDS."

During one of my conversations with Father Bill, I asked him to describe the creation process for these images. I had imagined him, a young priest whose days were filled by accompanying the sick and suffering, seeking to create art that helped them cope. After all, by this point I had heard several stories like the one Stephen told me about his prayer group in Toronto, in which Father Bill's art, which centered gay men with AIDS, sometimes even comparing their suffering to that of Jesus, offered hope and encouragement. But when I relayed this observation to Father Bill, he corrected me. His intended audience for his AIDS related art was actually not people with AIDS. Instead, he told me, his art was motivated partly by his anger. Some HIV and AIDS activists took to the streets; Father Bill headed to his studio. He wanted to hold up to society a mirror, in which individuals could see the callousness and empty indifference they displayed toward people with AIDS.

"I didn't do those pictures for people with AIDS; I did them for everybody else," he told me.

Regardless of his intent, Father Bill's art had an impact he never imagined, one that continues to reverberate all these decades later. He told me about his experience first hearing David Pais's story when he listened to my podcast, *Plague*. He repeated the story he had learned, about David's partner falling ill in the 1980s, David coming up to him after a healing Mass and asking if he had any kind of message for the dying man. Father Bill, David said, had suggested the image of the Virgin Mary setting up luminaria to guide his dying partner on his journey home. David's partner died just hours later, comforted by this image of Mary leading him to peace.

"The first time I heard the story about the luminaria, I broke down crying," Father Bill said.

Even thirty years later, Father Bill McNichols is still learning about the impact of his ministry. But for every story like Stephen's and David's, there are surely dozens more, individuals who were comforted by Father Bill's art or spiritual wisdom. We will never know the intimate details.

———

By 1989, Father Bill McNichols's ministry had taken a toll on him physically. He was worn out, the stress causing back spasms so severe he sought medical care. He had spent six years engaged in intense, personal ministry. His Jesuit superiors wanted him to take a break and enter the next phase of his formation. It wouldn't be easy for Father Bill to leave behind the relationships he had built in New York and the ministry that was still so tragically needed. But he agreed and packed up. He headed west and spent several months to retreat. By the end of 1990, he said goodbye to New York for good. His next chapter would be to study under a master iconographer and draw images that made their ways into churches all around the world.

Learning about Father Bill's coming out as a gay priest in the 1980s and then launching an AIDS ministry as a young Jesuit were the events that originally attracted me to his life story. When I learned that his work with HIV and AIDS ended in 1990, right before his relocation to New Mexico, I figured that would be the point at which I stopped documenting his life. But that turned out not to be the case. Father Bill has continued to make LGBT inclusion part of his ministry, even if it looks rather different from what he did in the 1980s.

Father Bill came out again in a very public way in 2002, when he was profiled in a *Time* magazine feature about gay priests. When he saw the story in the magazine, he was mortified.

In black and red block letters, the headline screamed: "Inside the church's closet." Next to that, a photo of Father Bill filled an entire page. It felt staged, with Bill's hands pressed together in prayer. And to clear up any confusion that the priest in the photo lived in the aforementioned closet, the first sentence of the story laid it all out: "The Rev. William Hart McNichols is gay." Father Bill said in the article that coming out was never easy, especially in a national magazine. But at that time, some leaders in the US church had scapegoated gay priests for the church's sexual abuse scandal. Bill found that intolerable.

"This is an extremely dangerous moment," he told *Time*.

Father Bill shared his story with the reporter under the impression that his voice would be one of many featured in the article. Strength in numbers.

"Talking to you is just as scary as the first time I came out to anyone," he told the reporter. "But you can't go through life hiding who you are and feel any honesty before God."

In the end, the report about the large number of gay priests in the church mentioned by name just him and two other openly gay priests, one of whom had left active ministry. Rather than joining a chorus of voices fighting against injustice, Father Bill was somewhat alone in pleading for compassion. He had never been one to hide his views on sexuality, but now his beliefs could be scrutinized by many, including those who held power over his ministry.

Father Bill had sometimes been at odds with his superiors for a few years—his independence and admittedly quirky behavior had generated long-simmering resentments between him and some high-level Jesuits—and attention from the article felt to Bill like it was the last straw. Father Bill said his superiors asked him to leave his ministry in New Mexico and move to a Jesuit community in St. Louis. He felt like they were asking him to give up too much. He told them he wasn't willing to relocate and said he would leave the order instead. His superiors didn't ask him to stay.

Separating from the Jesuits was a painful experience that Father Bill is uncomfortable discussing. He asked me several times to make sure that whatever I wrote about this part of his life wouldn't hurt his former religious brothers. He regards his seven years in AIDS ministry as a gift from the order and still professes a love for the Jesuits. Though he is no longer a Jesuit, Father Bill is still a Catholic priest in good standing. He lives in New Mexico and works full-time creating icons.

Father Bill told me he wants other gay Catholics to know that they have a place in the church. That's been the purpose of much of his life's work, and over the course of the friendship we've developed since I first emailed him, I've frequently reflected on his courage. I asked him during one of our conversations if he thought gay Catholics have an easier time today in the church than they did in the 1980s. It's not an easy question to answer. In 2005 and again in 2016, the Vatican effectively banned gay men from the priesthood. I've interviewed many LGBT people who have been fired from their jobs at Catholic schools and churches. Some gay Catholic groups are still being kicked out of parishes.

But I've also had the opportunity to tell these stories in part because of the Jesuits who publish the magazine where I write, including Father James Martin, a leader in ministry to LGBT Catholics, who gave me time and resources to travel and meet people like Father Bill. One of Father Bill's controversial AIDS crucifixion scenes even appeared on the cover of *America* magazine to help promote *Plague*. The place of gay Catholics in the church today is complicated. Father Bill listened to my question and thought for a moment before answering. Were things better today for gay Catholics? He wasn't sure. But he emphasized that he doesn't want to be portrayed as a victim. The shock therapy, the hate mail, the clash with his superiors. None of that was just or right, but Father Bill said his story doesn't feel particularly unique.

"Even today in the church, gay people don't have a green card. At any moment, you can be cut off," he told me. "And that has always been the way."

Father Bill is mild-mannered, and his gentle voice can paper over the strong images he invokes to describe the church's mistreatment of LGBT people. In a 2005 interview, he said the Vatican viewed gay people as "aberrations and mentally distorted" and treated them like "a group of heroin addicts." Fifteen years later, Father Bill has softened his language a bit. But it's clear he still feels hurt, both personally and on behalf of other LGBT Catholics who have been subjected to the church's cruelty. When I asked if he held any regrets about being open about his sexual orientation, he said no.

"Coming out has followed me and has been a source of persecution ever since I did it the first time," he said. He told me that a friend had shunned him after reading an article I had written for the *Washington Post* about his AIDS ministry, in which he was identified as a gay priest. "I can see why people don't want to do it, but I don't think I could have lived any other way. But it certainly didn't make living easy. It's been wonderful and difficult all at once."

Yet in spite of all that persecution and pain, he sees his life and ministry as a gift.

"To have that many days, seven years of intimate relationships with people, talks with people about things that they would never tell anybody else," he told me, "it was everything I ever wanted to be as a priest."

———

About a year after I first met Father Bill, I hung a medal around my neck, the one that I reflected on while writing at the coffee shop in Boystown. It's small, about an inch tall and half as wide. It's sterling silver, made in Italy. The kind of trinket you can find in cathedral gift shops. On the front is the profile of Aloysius Gonzaga, the saint who gave up a life of privilege for one of prayer and poverty. In 1591, a plague broke out in Rome. Aloysius volunteered at a Jesuit hospital, even after he was forbidden from visiting the ill because his own health was at risk. Eventually, he too caught the plague, dying at age twenty-three. Saint Aloysius has become the patron saint of those living with HIV and AIDS today.

Many Catholics turn to the saints for comfort, inspiration, and sometimes even divine help. Father Bill thinks of them as friends and companions. I admit I found it jarring at first when he spoke about the saints as if they were present and active in his life. Upon further reflection, I realized my reaction was driven, in part, by the reality that the saints have not been a source of spiritual solace for me. I think in many ways I was unable to identify with their lives. For much of my own, I've occupied a space on the margins of the church. Admittedly, part of this is my own doing. By standing in the figurative doorway, I can easily leave whenever I feel threatened. But that liminal faith is also the product of worrying that I am indeed not fully welcome, that my identity as a gay man somehow makes me anathema to the faith. Saints are like the superheroes of the church, surely too far inside the institution for me to see from the space I occupy near the exit. Father Bill's history with Saint Aloysius changed my perspective.

I bought the Aloysius medal because I wanted help in telling the stories of people who lived and worked during the AIDS epidemic. It turns out that Father Bill's artwork had helped tie Aloysius to HIV and AIDS. He was among the first people to depict the Italian saint caring for victims of this new plague. There's an ad in a June 1987 issue of Dignity's newsletter with one of Father Bill's drawings, depicting Aloysius visiting a man in a hospital bed, letting readers know they could purchase his HIV and AIDS-related artwork to use in their own ministries. The image of Aloysius as the patron saint of people with AIDS seemed to stick, and a former head of the Jesuits had even urged the Vatican to make the association official (though I've been unable to discover what, if anything, happened to that request).

If Father Bill hadn't been honest with himself and others, it's possible he never would have engaged in the ministry that provided solace to David and Stephen and many others like them, whose stories we'll never know. That's partly why I wear the Aloysius medal. As a gay Catholic, it makes me feel connected to the pioneers who came before me, to people like Father Bill.

Epilogue

New York

After Mass, I head downstairs to the church hall. The first few minutes before delivering any talk are always the worst for me. I panic, wondering if anyone will show up. Then I develop a sort of dry-mouth condition, requiring constant refills of little plastic cups of water. Which then makes me worry about the location of the nearest bathroom. I fumble with the handwritten notes I've prepared, wondering if I should have printed out the full text instead. In between all the worrying, I try my best to make small talk with either the host or those few wonderful souls who arrive early. It's only when groups of people start trickling in that my nerves subside and I remember that, despite the sweating and the dry mouth, I actually enjoy doing this. I take a couple of deep breaths and remind myself that these are friendly audiences who want to hear what I have to say. Tonight will be no different.

On this particular evening, I'm in the basement hall of the Church of Saint Paul the Apostle, just a short walk from Columbus Circle in New York. I'm there to talk about my podcast that has recently debuted, chronicling a few of the stories now included in this book. The series, produced by the Jesuit magazine *America*, where I write about the church, has received a fair bit of positive media coverage, even earning a recommendation in the *New York Times* and a feature on NPR. But it was the hundreds of heartfelt, and often deeply personal, emails and messages sent to me from listeners all around the world that have made the most impact. Some were from people in their sixties and seventies, recalling how they responded, or didn't, during the height of the HIV crisis, or telling me about loved ones who had died from AIDS. Others were from LGBT people and long-term HIV survivors who said they appreciated that people like them were finally given space to tell their stories—and by a Catholic publication no less.

One message in particular stood out to me and I think of it often: "Hi! I wanted to say your podcast has been such a blessing for me as a gay Black Catholic who is not out to my family yet. I'm learning so much and my fears about myself are going away and you have inspired me!"

That had been my goal from the beginning, to help young LGBT Catholics, along with their family and friends, lean on this history, *our* history, to dispel fear. After fighting to bring these stories to a wider audience, I felt validated hearing that the hard work was paying off. This listener and I stayed in touch for a bit, and I learned more about his story. He had been raised in a Baptist home and discovered he was gay while in high school. He struggled to reconcile his sexuality with his faith. He thought he could use prayer to fight off his attraction to other men but eventually realized that the "pray away the gay" method was just making him miserable. He stopped. But he wanted to continue to have a faith life and he eventually found a home in the Catholic Church. That wasn't perfect either, he soon discovered. And that's where the stories of Sister Carol, Father Bill, David Pais, and others came in.

"Everyone has a story, especially the LGBT community of which I am a part. I love that this is being discussed in your podcast because it's like there is a culture of don't-ask-don't-tell in the church right now," he wrote to me. "I'm being liberated by your podcast."

That liberation came at a cost. A sadness seems to accompany many of the people I interviewed for this book, though it's not anything I can quite put my finger on. Father Bill came closest to articulating what I intuited when he told me he sees a collective sense of shame about how society responded to HIV and AIDS. Most people would rather not think about those dark days.

When I started reporting this project, my motivation was in many ways selfish. I struggled with my decision to remain Catholic while knowing the institution didn't embrace me fully as a gay man. While I have been fortunate that many of my experiences in the church have been fulfilling, there have been challenges. Had I known about the work of Father Bill and Sister Carol, perhaps those moments wouldn't have caused so much grief.

Even as we made the *Plague* podcast, it became clear what a fraught issue homosexuality remains in the church. We agonized over how much of my personal life should be included, fearful that identifying myself as gay would limit the audience or provoke backlash. Ultimately, we decided the series just didn't make sense if I wasn't honest about why I found creating it to be so important to me personally. Even the hate mail that eventually arrived, both in my inbox and, more alarmingly, to my home, did not cause me to regret my decision to be truthful.

Years after I first spoke to Carol, I reported on another story involving LGBT people and the Catholic Church. In the fall of 2020, video footage surfaced in a documentary about Pope Francis, in which he says he supports the notion of civil unions for same-sex couples. Though the pope didn't change church teaching, the intense interest in his words signaled the hunger among LGBT Catholics for any words of affirmation from church leaders.

After I reported the news, I was invited to offer commentary on several national and international television programs. Whereas I once would have agonized about commenting on stories that touch on homosexuality and the church, like back when I hid behind poll numbers and official statements during the debate over same-sex marriage, I had no such fear when anchors asked me how LGBT Catholics greeted the news about civil unions. I answered honestly and directly, nowhere near as fearful that my own dual identities could become public. Without having spent years researching this book, I'm not certain I would have been so willing to speak openly. Thinking back on this experience, some words Carol's New York friend Jim D'Eramo told me during one of our interviews came to mind.

"Without your history, you don't have an identity."

Knowing this history helped edify me again a few months later, when the Vatican's doctrinal office released a statement in early 2021 reminding priests that they cannot bless same-sex unions. The statement says flatly that God "does not and cannot bless sin."

I considered my own longing to remain part of this church, in which the sacraments that sustained my ancestors connect me today to believers throughout the world. To balance that desire with a love I know to be sacred has not always been easy. The stories I've learned help me make sense of this new challenge, and at the same time, I look toward the future, seeking out voices who speak prophetically about the day when Jesus's commandment that we love one another will be a step closer toward fulfillment.

One of those voices belongs to Father Bryan Massingale, perhaps best known today for his advocacy around racial justice. He credits the vantage point that comes from being African American in a church in which fewer than 5 percent of its members identify as Black for his ability to recognize and call out injustice that might otherwise go unchallenged.

A pair of grieving parents had approached him in 1983, just a few months after his ordination, and explained that their son, only in his twenties, had died from AIDS. They requested a funeral for him, but they asked him not to acknowledge their son's sexual orientation or his cause of death during the Mass. Not wanting to compound their grief, he agreed.

But the day of the funeral, when he gazed out into the congregation, he saw that half the crowd appeared to be gay men. Friends of the deceased, perhaps a partner, all grieving. He felt trapped, complicit in perpetuating stigma that he knew had no place in a Christian community.

"We have to do better," he said.

Unlike Father Bill McNichols, who suspected that he would be labeled a gay priest because of his work in HIV and AIDS, Father Massingale harbored no such worries. In the Catholic settings where he lectured and preached, "it was almost like Black gays didn't even exist," he said. That meant he could minister to gay couples affected by HIV and teach seminarians about AIDS ministry without worrying what others thought about his sexual orientation, a veneer of racism helping him keep a secret he wasn't yet ready to share with the world.

As a young Black priest fighting racism in the 1980s, he felt compelled to highlight how the stigma associated with HIV and AIDS is another form of unjust discrimination. Later, as one of just a few openly gay priests, he pushed the Black Catholic community to take the epidemic more seriously and he challenged fellow theologians to address more robustly the impact of HIV and AIDS on communities of color.

His words continue to challenge today. The church will not be just, he said recently, until LGBT Catholics feel that we can "confidently and insistently proclaim that we are equally redeemed by Christ and radically loved by God."

———

As I finished this project, I paused to think of how I was able to capture but a fraction of the many worthy stories from our history. Part of that was simply the limitations that accompany writing a book, but there was also the passage of time. From the moment I spoke to Carol, it was clear that time was not on our side. She was advancing in years and many of her stories involved Sister Mary Ellen. A natural second step for me to learn more about their time in New York would be to interview her, but she died in 2014. I had missed my chance. This pattern played out repeatedly over the next few years. Nearly everyone I interviewed in New York told me I had to learn more about Sister Patrice Murphy, the legendary Sister of Charity at Saint Vincent's. But she was too ill to speak to me when I first reached out in 2016 and she passed away a few years later. So much of her story has now been lost.

This race against time came into sharp focus for me during the production of the podcast. My producer, Eloise Blondiau, and I had interviewed a number of nurses and sisters associated with Saint Vincent's. We met many of them during a chaotic week in New York in the summer of 2019.

In order to help us understand the culture of the hospital before the dramatic protest by ACT UP, we contacted a retired surgeon, Dr. Christopher Mills, who agreed to trek into our midtown studio from New Jersey. Following the interview, during which he told us about the hospital's culture in the 1990s, Eloise and I walked him to the door. We thanked him and his wife for making time to be interviewed, and he pulled me aside.

"Thank you for what you're doing," he said. He explained that though he and his wife were Catholic, their children had struggled with the church, including one who is gay. "I'm glad you're helping to tell this story."

Just a few weeks later, I received an email from one of our contacts at the Sisters of Charity telling us that Dr. Mills had died. Our interview with him had been his last. The sisters asked if they could have a copy of the audio for their archives, to help tell the full story of Saint Vincent's.

———

Back at my talk in New York in 2020, with the start of another epidemic unknowingly just days away, I scan the crowd. Mostly gay and mostly older, men who had been roughly my age now back in 1985. This was calming in one sense, because it meant they cared about the topic of my talk. But it also meant they knew firsthand the horrors of living through the height of the HIV and AIDS crisis, compounded by the assault from church leaders on the gay community at the time. What on earth could I tell them that they didn't already know far more viscerally than I could ever understand? And then I saw a face I recognized: David Pais. The sweating and dry mouth returned. I gulped down a few sips of water before walking over to say hello.

"David!" I said. "You didn't have to come to this, but it's great to see you."

A few months earlier, he had finished a grueling pilgrimage in Spain, fulfilling a promise he made in 1994 to honor people who had died from AIDS. During a stop in one of the churches that line the route, he was struck by a crucifix that depicted Christ covered in purple welts. His mind went straight to the KS lesions that covered the body of his partner, memories that still haunt him decades later. He was also just a couple of months away from retiring from the Gay Men's Health Crisis. I told him that his story would be part of my talk that night and that I hoped I would do it justice. He told me not to worry.

For the next forty minutes, I recounted some of the stories that are now part of this book. I recalled statistics that show HIV and AIDS are not a thing of the past, but an ongoing fight that continues to affect communities of color hardest and that deserves more attention and resources. The reaction from the crowd was encouraging and their inquiries thoughtful. When I answered the final question, the host thanked me and gifted me a tank top with a print of Saint Aloysius Gonzaga on the front, meant to be worn during an upcoming AIDS charity bike ride I planned to complete.

After the event, David thanked me for sharing part of his life with others and for introducing him to similar stories he hadn't previously known. We said goodbye, and I noticed a group of young adults had assembled nearby. I smiled and walked over, my nerves from before the talk now well under control. I actually love these moments, when I transform into reporter mode. Tell me your name, your age, where you're from—and a little bit of your story. I learned they were part of the parish's LGBT group, Out at Saint Paul's. Each of them was in their twenties. We chatted for another minute or so, and as I prepared to excuse myself to meet my husband and some friends for a celebratory dinner, one of the guys in the group looked at me.

"Thanks for your work," he said. "We hadn't known any of that history. It's good to know we're not alone."

Acknowledgments

This book culminates five years' worth of research into the Catholic Church's response to HIV and AIDS. Its completion was made possible because of the many people who offered support, insight, and a steady stream of encouragement.

Thank you to my literary agent Roger Freet at Folio Literary Management, who stuck by this project for many years, to Lil Copan and her team at Broadleaf Books for taking a chance on my idea, to Jana Riess for her tireless, expert, and thoughtful editing, and to Heidi Hill for her fact checking.

Some of the material in this book is based on interviews used in my podcast *Plague: Untold Stories of AIDS and the Catholic Church*, produced in 2019 by America Media. I am grateful to my many colleagues at *America* who invested time, space, and resources into the project, especially Sebastian Gomes, as well as Ken Arko, Vivian Cabrera, Glenda Castro, Zac Davis, Alison Hamilton, Traug Keller, Matt Malone, SJ, Lisa Manico, Ashley McKinless, Tucker Redding, SJ, Nick Sawicki, Sam Sawyer, SJ, Robert David Sullivan, Eric Sundrup, SJ, Shawn Tripoli, Maggi Van Dorn, and Kerry Weber. Colleen Dulle graciously volunteered her reporting skills to help tell the story of Bethany Place and Joe Hoover, SJ, allowed me to crash his writing workshop to sharpen my prose.

Thank you to Mark McDermott and Yuval David, and members of the Raskob Foundation, for supporting the project and Kelly Hughes for introducing the series to a wider audience. A special word of thanks to Timothy Reidy for giving me the flexibility to work on this book and to James Martin, SJ, for having faith in my ability to tell these stories, for his invaluable ministry that has consoled countless LGBT Catholics and their families, and for regularly making me laugh even during the most stressful points in completing this project.

Plague would never have been possible without the tireless work of Eloise Blondiau, whose patience, tenacity, and innate storytelling ability helped create a series that moved more than a few people to tears. I am also indebted to Eloise for helping to recraft some stories from *Plague* for this book, transforming the energy we captured in audio into compelling text.

To the hundreds of listeners who messaged me to share their own stories about HIV and AIDS, thank you. You helped me better understand this complex time in our history and I hope you saw reflected in this book some of your own insights and thoughts.

My work benefited from the expertise of a number of institutions, including the Gerber/Hart Library and Archives in Chicago, Loyola University Chicago, the Catholic Worker Collection at Marquette University, the University of Notre Dame, the ACT UP Oral History Project, Most Holy Redeemer Parish in San Francisco, Bethany Place, the Sisters of Charity of New York, the National Catholic Reporter, Out at St. Paul, the Paulist Center, New Ways Ministry, Dignity USA, the Archdiocese of Washington, and the Catholic Health Association.

Many people took time to answer questions, make connections, and provide information, and I am grateful to Dr. Daniel Baxter, Jason Berry, Terri Cook, Francis DeBernardo, David France, Jon Fuller, SJ, Jim Hubbard, Father Pat Lee, Father Matt Link, Stephen Martz, Carl Meirose, Stephen P. Millies, Elena Miranda, Dean Ogren, Nicole Pascarelli O'Brien, Anthony Petro, Phillip Runkel, Thomas Rzeznik, Roger Schlueter, Carl Siciliano, Jeffrey Stone, Chris Summa, Pete Toms, and Vinita Wright. I owe a special word of thanks to the many reporters who chronicled the early days of the HIV and AIDS crisis in real time, especially at LGBT newspapers, whose work helped immensely with this project.

A number of friends and colleagues provided vital encouragement, assistance, introductions, and feedback over the past few years. I am indebted to Michael Bayer, Bob Bordone, Matt Collette, Justin DeJong, Elizabeth Dias, Donal Godfrey, SJ, Josh Kaplan, Alexia Kelley, Father Frank Latzko, Tobin Low, Dell Miller, Joe Nuzzi, Kerry Robinson, Thomas Rosica, CSB, Michael Ruzicki, James Shed, Stephen Staten, Olga Segura, Adam Teicholz, Father Michael Trail, and Michael Vazquez. And a special thanks to my family, James and Nancy O'Loughlin, Megan O'Loughlin, Brent Laurin, and Kathryn O'Loughlin for their generous encouragement and support.

Matthew Sitman was instrumental in helping me formulate ideas in the early stages of this book; Kaya Oakes graciously introduced me to Broadleaf Books; Anna Marchese taught me how to record compelling audio; Christopher White read draft after draft, even when I should have spent a fair bit more time polishing them; and William Critchley-Menor, SJ, provided valuable feedback during the long days preparing my final draft.

My goal in writing this book was to do justice to stories of heroism that have not been told. Dozens of people spent time with me sharing stories from decades ago that are in many cases still visibly painful. Thank you especially to Father William Hart McNichols, Carol Baltosiewich, and David Pais, each of whom responded promptly to my countless telephone calls, text messages, and emails with thoughtful answers to what I repeatedly promised was just one more follow-up question.

A quick word of thanks to the baristas at Intelligentsia in Chicago, for brewing coffee during a pandemic and providing a comfortable space to work outside in the summer of 2020.

I am so thankful to my husband, Dr. Matthew R. Klein, for helping me to understand the medical issues associated with HIV and AIDS, for his insightful and encouraging feedback, and for his seemingly limitless reservoir of support and good humor, even during my most mania-filled days when trying to meet deadlines. Thank you.

Finally, the battle against HIV is ongoing. Annually, tens of thousands of people are diagnosed with HIV in the United States and many more around the world. In 1986, Dignity published an AIDS prayer in its newsletter that remains as relevant today:

"Bless those who care for the sick, and hasten the discovery of a cure."
Amen.

Notes

1: Time Was of the Essence

9 *"When my story was published"*: Michael O'Loughlin, "Being Gay at a Catholic University," *Religion & Politics*, June 18, 2013, https://tinyurl.com/tm63zdkh.

10 *"the pope's comments provided hope"*: Michael O'Loughlin, "Pope Surprises on Women, Gays, Marriage," Religion News Service, July 29, 2013, https://tinyurl.com/38ad63u7.

10 *"Andrew Sullivan, another gay Catholic"*: Andrew Sullivan, "Francis' Sunlight: Reax," The Dish, July 29, 2013, https://tinyurl.com/4tf7cm6s.

10 *"unfair to ban gay groups"*: Michael O'Loughlin, "In Boston, an Ugly St. Patrick's Day Tradition Continues," *The Advocate*, March 10, 2014, https://tinyurl.com/scxnpdr5.

11 *"urging the pope to speak out"*: Michael O'Loughlin, "Francis's Papal Bull," *Foreign Policy*, April 1, 2014, https://tinyurl.com/hp6673js.

11 *"effectively banned gay teachers"*: Michael O'Loughlin, "As Societal Norms Change, Catholic Groups Enforce the Rules," Crux, December 5, 2014, https://tinyurl.com/2b96t8cs.

11 *"I interviewed transgender Catholics"*: Michael O'Loughlin, "Transgender Catholics Hope to Build Bridges in the Church," Crux, March 7, 2016, https://tinyurl.com/2hz3au68.

15 *"more than 362,000 of them died"*: "HIV/AIDS: Snapshots of an Epidemic," amfAR, The Foundation for AIDS Research, https://tinyurl.com/hm6w8vhk. The numbers of deaths reported in subsequent pages come from this timeline, unless otherwise noted.

2: "Through Their Own Fault"

18 *"memorials were relatively rare"*: Greg Cook, "How do we honor those lost to AIDS? From the AIDS Quilt to new memorials," WBUR, May 1, 2015.

18 *"one of the nation's first AIDS memorials"*: Interview of Andrew Berman by Anna Marchese, July 2017.

22 *"they were almost always deadly"*: "What Are HIV and AIDS?," HIV.gov, available at https://tinyurl.com/w8zab3tf.

22 *"The case numbers were dramatic"*: "HIV/AIDS: Snapshots of an Epidemic," https://tinyurl.com/v9vfawhd.

23 *"A third of Americans believed sex between gay people should be illegal"*: George Skelton, "The Times Poll: U.S. Voters in No Mood to Launch Moral Crusade," *Los Angeles Times*, July 20, 1986, https://tinyurl.com/y2nd3nk4.

24 *"We're not going to take that chance"*: Larry McShane, "Archdiocese Backtracks on Shelter for AID [*sic*] Students," Associated Press, August 31, 1985.

24 *"Jesus Christ is there"*: Larry Rohter, "Pastor Scolds Parish for Rejecting an AIDS Shelter," *New York Times*, September 2, 1985, https://tinyurl.com/jjauc5as.

25 *"one badass nun"*: Author interview with Dr. Daniel Baxter, October 19, 2017. Baxter writes about his working relationship with Sister Pascal Conforti in *The Least of These My Brethren* (New York: Harmony Books, 1997).

25 *"the love she saw in the hospital"*: Pascal Conforti, OSU, "A View from the Edge," *America*, December 6, 1997.

26 *"one lifetime perhaps isn't enough"*: Neal Hirschfeld, "The Gift of Love," *New York Daily News*, November 22, 1998. And author interview with Pascal Conforti, September 21, 2017.

26 *"The reporters laughed again"*: See the 2015 short film *When AIDS Was Funny*, by Scott Calonico, available at "The Reagan Administration's Unearthed Response to the AIDS Crisis Is Chilling," *Vanity Fair*, December 1, 2015, https://tinyurl.com/53y6fn3e.

26 *"six years into the crisis"*: Hank Plante, "Reagan's Legacy," San Francisco AIDS Foundation, February 10, 2011, available at https://tinyurl.com/64bm2ea2. Reagan first addressed AIDS at a press conference in 1985. See Philip Boffey, "Reagan Defends Financing for AIDS," *New York Times*, September 18, 1985, https://tinyurl.com/73p3ea9u.

3: Hospital Sisters

36 *"about three hundred thousand Americans had been living with HIV,"* "HIV and AIDS Timeline," Centers for Disease Control and Prevention. https://npin.cdc .gov/pages/hiv-and-aids-timeline.

37 *"volunteered its tax-exempt status":* "History," SAVE Inc., https://tinyurl.com/ fkx58w93, retrieved August 23, 2020.

38 *"They couldn't wait to get home to shower":* Roger Schlueter, "Nuns Reach Out to People with AIDS," *Belleville News-Democrat,* October 28, 1988.

39 *"which served primarily gay men":* Sari Staver, "Former Chicagoan Bob Rybicki Dies," *Windy City Times,* September 10, 2016, https://tinyurl.com/yp8nsv9t. Rybicki would eventually be received into the Episcopal Church, marry his husband, and become a leader in HIV and AIDS care in San Francisco.

39 *"Was this person gay, promiscuous, a drug user?":* Michael Hirsley, "Victims of More Than Just AIDS," *Chicago Tribune,* April 13, 1990, https://tinyurl.com/ vvdnrhu7.

4: "It Has to Be a Gay Person"

46 *"draft exemption status":* "Draft Refusal," photo, *St. Louis Post-Dispatch,* July 2, 1971; "Priest Hails Antidraft Seminarians," *St. Louis Post-Dispatch,* July 16, 1971.

46 *"Dignity . . . invited priests to celebrate Mass":* "Dignity USA History," Dignity, https://www.dignityusa.org/history, accessed August 23, 2020.

48 *"You can't be afraid of this":* Bob Reilly, "Homosexual and Catholic," *St. Anthony Messenger,* July 1984.

48 *"Omaly would die from AIDS-related complications":* Mills Roger Omaly, Dartmouth University alumni obituary, accessed August 26, 2020, https://tinyurl .com/7z6ea4fc.

49 *"At the end of Mass":* "AIDS Victims Attend Special Catholic Mass," *National Catholic Reporter,* October 14, 1983.

51 *"Sister Patrice Murphy, who was a fierce advocate":* For more on Sister Patrice, see Thomas F. Rzeznik, "The Church and the AIDS Crisis in New York City," *U.S. Catholic Historian,* vol. 34, no. 1, Winter 2016, 143–65.

53 *"The church will come around":* Robert Massa, "Vows of Silence, Priests with AIDS," written for *the Village Voice,* published in the *San Francisco Examiner,* March 29, 1987.

54 *"We have to bring healing to each other":* James A. Revson, "A Mission to Heal," *Newsday,* December 22, 1987.

54 *"suggested gay Catholics try to 'switch'":* John May, "The Tube," *St. Louis Review,* May 29, 1987.

5: CATHOLIC TO THE BONES

60 *"in all capital letters.":* Lawrence K. Altman, "Rare Cancer Seen in 41 Homosexuals," *New York Times,* July 3, 1981, https://tinyurl.com/4zc7s7xv.

62 *"More than a hundred people called that first night":* "History," Gay Men's Health Crisis (GMHC), https://www.gmhc.org/history, retrieved August 23, 2020.

62 *"sizable donation":* Author interview with Andy Humm, October 19, 2017.

6: "AN INTRINSIC MORAL EVIL"

67 *"Saint Francis Xavier Church":* See Rzeznik, "The Church and the AIDS Crisis," 159. He notes that Dignity's New York chapter had struggled to find a suitable place to meet for worship and for six years used a Jesuit residence offered to them by Father John J. McNeill, but quickly outgrew the chapel. When Saint Francis Xavier agreed to host the Masses, church leaders, fearful of negative repercussions, asked them not to print the name or address of the church on flyers.

67 *"the church's crackdown on gay and lesbian activism":* "History," https://www.dignityusa.org/history.

68 *"they can be changed":* Ari L. Goldman, "Homosexual Group Holds Its Final Mass," *New York Times,* March 9, 1987, https://tinyurl.com/fxx6s3p3.

68 *"Worshippers stood on their kneelers and cheered":* Goldman, "Homosexual Group."

69 *"so angry at church leaders":* *The Boy Who Found Gold: A Journey into the Art and Spirit of William Hart McNichols,* DVD, dir. Christopher Summa (Dramaticus Films, 2016).

69 *"Pope John Paul II had not publicly addressed HIV or AIDS":* Robert Suro, "Vatican and the AIDS Fight: Amid Worry, Papal Reticence," *New York Times,* January 29, 1988, https://tinyurl.com/8pk4dzhc.

70 *"written in English":* Bruce Buursma, "Vatican Targets U.S. in Blast at Homosexuality," *Chicago Tribune,* October 31, 1986, https://tinyurl.com/29vazxky.

70 *"why ban the natural expression of that gift?"*: See John J. McNeill, *The Church and the Homosexual* (London: Sheed Andrews and McMeel, 1976). Further reading in Richard L. Smith, *AIDS, Gays, and the American Catholic Church* (Cleveland: Pilgrim Press, 1994).

70 *"an 'intrinsic moral evil'"*: "Letter to the Bishops of the Catholic Church on the Pastoral Care of Homosexual Persons," The Holy See, October 1, 1986, https://tinyurl.com/28x2syuj.

71 *"US bishops had actively preached against this kind of violence"*: As early as 1985, Cardinal Joseph Bernardin of Chicago told the Illinois Gay and Lesbian Task Force in a letter that "there is no place for arbitrary discrimination and prejudice against a person because of sexual attraction." He even suggested that he could see Catholics supporting civil rights measures for gays and lesbians if they didn't contradict church teaching. Still, bishops across the country were fighting bills that would have extended gay civil rights and the church was increasingly losing. In New York, earlier in the year, the city council passed a gay rights bill over the objections of the church. See "NY Cardinal Condemns Gay Violence," Dignity USA, September 1988.

71 *"Gay Catholics were outraged"*: Dignity, Inc., Newsletter, Dec. 1986–Jan. 1987.

7: Saint Vincent's

75 *"a history as colorful as"*: Michael J. O'Loughlin, "The Catholic Hospital That Pioneered AIDS Care," *America*, January 24, 2020, https://tinyurl.com/ekabtunj

77 *"a graduate of a Catholic high school"*: Alex Vadukul, "Patrick O'Connell, 67, Dies; Raised Awareness of AIDS With Art," *New York Times*, May 3, 2021.

79 *"The archdiocese opened their arms"*: Author interview with Dr. Ramon Torres, July 24, 2019.

80 *"the first in his family to go to college"*: David France, "Another AIDS Casualty," profile of Torres in *New York* magazine, April 4, 2008, https://nymag.com/news/features/45785/.

80 *"young, robust, muscular gay men from the Village literally dying"*: Ronald Bayer and Gerald M. Oppenheimer, eds., *AIDS Doctors: Voices from the Front Lines* (New York: Oxford University Press, 2000), 38.

81 *"Dr. Torres was featured"*: Bruce Lambert, "Study Finds Alarming AIDS Rate in Homeless Shelter," *New York Times*, June 5, 1989, https://tinyurl.com/54439yk8.

82 *"because of these trials"*: David France, New York magazine.

82 *"at the hospital's AIDS hospice"*: Beth Nichol, "In Memoriam: Sister M. Patrice Murphy, SC," Sisters of Charity of New York, April 19, 2019, https://tinyurl.com/25ubv3fe.

83 *"tried to make patients smile"*: "St. Vincent's Remembered," *Out*, August 17, 2010, https://tinyurl.com/2hempfn4.

83 *"classically trained pianist"*: Author interview with Joan Blanchfield, July 9, 2019.

84 *"closeted priest from Philadelphia"*: Author interview with Dr. Torres, January 10, 2021.

8: LETTER OF THE LAW

85 *"He spoke out on social justice issues often"*: For more on Cardinal O'Connor, see Steven Greenhouse, "Union Celebrates O'Connor's Labor Views," *New York Times*, July 24, 2000, https://tinyurl.com/2erbsxny; and Brianne Korn, "N.Y. Cardinal Was Fierce Foe of Anti-Semitism," *Jewish Telegraphic Agency*, May 5, 2000.

86 *"pleaded with doctors"*: Michael Specter, "Koop Asks Doctors to Back Condom Use," *Washington Post*, October 13, 1987, https://tinyurl.com/f48d5zdy/.

87 *"a very grave mistake"*: Ari L. Goldman, "Cardinal Won't Allow Instruction on Condoms in Programs on AIDS," *New York Times*, December 14, 1987, https://tinyurl.com/y64hbnbf.

88 *"The committee's work"*: "Bishops Set Up Task Force to Tackle AIDS Problem," *Chicago Sun-Times*, June 13, 1987.

88 *"released statements on the epidemic"*: Daniel J. Lehmann, "Bernardin Urges AIDS 'Care, Compassion,'" *Chicago Sun-Times*, October 24, 1986. The cardinal was aware of the pending Vatican letter and sought to lessen the blow to the gay community by releasing his own letter ahead of time. Bernardin's letter, "A Challenge and a Responsibility: A Pastoral Statement on the Church's Response to the AIDS Crisis," served as a framework for "The Many Faces of AIDS."

88 *"a growing national emergency"*: Author interview with Fr. Michael Place, August 12, 2020.

88 *"How could the church contribute"*: Author interview with Fr. Michael Place, August 12, 2020.

88 *"The bishops felt they had achieved their elusive goal"*: Goldman, "Cardinal Won't Allow Instruction on Condoms."

88 *"lashed out at gay men"*: Daniel J. Lehmann, "Bishops Take Stand on AIDS—Back Condom Education, if . . . ," *Chicago Sun-Times*, December 11, 1987.

89 *"condemned public health campaigns"*: "The Many Faces of AIDS," National Conference of Catholic Bishops Administrative Board, December 7, 1987, https://tinyurl.com/3nhnz7au.

90 *"not on his fellow cardinal, but on the media"*: Goldman, "Cardinal Won't Allow Instruction on Condoms."

91 *"Cardinal Law said in a joint statement"*: "N.E. Prelates against AIDS Condom Use," Associated Press, December 14, 1987.

91 *"did not endorse the use of condoms"*: Anthony M. Petro, *After the Wrath of God: AIDS, Sexuality, and American Religion* (New York: Oxford University Press, 2015), 126.

91 *"he did irreparable harm"*: "Weakland Cites O'Connor," Dignity, Inc. Newsletter, March 1988.

91 *"universal doctrine of the church"*: Agosteno Bono, "Vatican Letter," *Pittsburgh Catholic*, November 1, 1991.

92 *"unacceptable from the moral aspect"*: "Pope Addresses American 'Condom' Document," Dignity, Inc. Newsletter, June 1988.

92 *"urged the bishops not to rescind"*: Peter Steinfels, "Catholic Bishops Vote to Retain Controversial Statement on AIDS," *New York Times*, June 28, 1988, https://tinyurl.com/59vdt9x.

92 *"he asked the group to draft a new letter"*: "Faces of Bishops," Dignity, Inc. Newsletter, July/August 1988.

92 *"the press often focused on church leaders"*: Diane Winston, "'Shame, Fear, and Compassion': Media Coverage of Catholicism during the First Decade of the AIDS Crisis," in *In the Lógos of Love: Promise and Predicament in Catholic Intellectual Life*, edited by Fr. James L. Heft, SM, and Una M. Cadegan (New York: Oxford University Press, 2016), 171–94.

93 *"worked at Saint Vincent's"*: Author interview with Sister Karen Helfenstein, July 9, 2019.

94 *"kept condoms hidden in their desks"*: Mireya Navarro, "Ethics of Giving AIDS Advice Troubles Catholic Hospitals," *New York Times*, January 3, 1993, https://tinyurl.com/2cabas5r.

95 *"The group had formed in 1987"*: "ACT UP Accomplishments: 1987–2012," https://actupny.com/actions/.

95 *"Security guards were being abusive"*: Gerri Wells, "ACT UP Oral History Project," interview 075 by Sarah Schulman, May 24, 2007, https://tinyurl.com/wm4x5f6u.

96 *"Darren was furious"*: "Adding Insult to Injury," *OutWeek*, September 18, 1989, 13, https://tinyurl.com/3ekbz7e6.

97 *"out of earshot of patients"*: Author interview with Dr. Mills, July 10, 2019.

97 *"the community it served"*: Neil Broome, "ACT UP Oral History Project," interview 055 by Sarah Schulman, April 25, 2004, https://tinyurl.com/53mkzncv.

9: "Stop the Church"

99 *"had been chaotic"*: Sarah Schulman, *Let the Record Show: A Political History of ACT UP New York, 1987–1993* (New York: Farrar, Straus and Giroux, 2021).

100 *"The archdiocese . . . sued in 1984"*: Josh Barbanel, "Archbishop Challenges Koch's Order on Hiring," *New York Times*, November 27, 1984, https://tinyurl.com/wcuu2ucf.

100 *"blocked gay Catholics from protesting"*: "Koch, at Gay Pride Parade, Reaffirms Support for NYC Gay Rights Bill," Associated Press, July 1, 1985.

100 *"campaign against a gay civil rights bill"*: Charles W. Bell, "O'C Seeks Help against Gay Bill," *New York Daily News*, January 11, 1986.

100 *"pressured the city into promoting abstinence"*: Marcia Kramer, "AIDS Afflicts 40 Teens Here," *New York Daily News*, November 11, 1987.

100 *"refused to reconsider his ban on Dignity"*: "Homosexual Group Ban Will Not Be Lifted, O'Connor Says," UPI, February 8, 1988.

100 *"a revolt, a rebellion, a resistance."*: Schulman, *Let the Record Show*, 137.

100 *"before his death from AIDS in 1990"*: Liz Fields, "Facing Death from AIDS, Keith Haring Kept Creating," *American Masters*, PBS, November 19, 2020, https://tinyurl.com/tnxkmvkw.

101 *"7 percent of the respondents . . . were still practicing"*: The religion scholar Anthony Petro reports on this study in his excellent book *After the Wrath of God* (New York: Oxford University Press, 2015), 146.

102 *"I tried reciting the Catholic prayers"*: Sean Strub, *Body Counts: A Memoir of Politics, Sex, AIDS, and Survival* (New York: Scribner, 2014), 165.

103 *"gentle recognition of our relationship"*: Strub, *Body Counts*, 214.

103 *"some internal debate"*: Kim Masters, "Here Is 'the Church,'" *Washington Post*, August 14, 1991, https://tinyurl.com/pju82km8.

103 *"claim that condoms were ineffective in fighting AIDS"*: "Vatican Meeting Hears O'Connor Assail Condom Use," AP, November 14, 1989. O'Connor joined other New York bishops in 1992 in stating that the failure rate of condoms could be compared to "giving our children a cereal that caused death 17 percent of the time," as reported in "NY Bishops Condemn Condom Distribution," Catholic News Service, November 27, 1992.

103 *"planned to remain outside"*: Victor Mendolia, "ACT UP Oral History Project," interview 097 by Sarah Schulman, August 15, 2008, https://tinyurl.com/ew5ubfvx.

104 *"murderous AIDS policy"*: Vincent Gagliostro, "ACT UP Oral History Project," interview 064 by Sarah Schulman, July 8, 2005, https://tinyurl.com/2uvke965.

104 *"murderous AIDS policy"*: Schulman, *Let the Record Show*, 152.

106 *"May the Lord bless the man I love"*: Strub, *Body Counts*, 230.

108 *"you've got to listen"*: Author interview with Dr. Anthony Fauci, May 26, 2020.

109 *"the ads frustrated public health experts"*: Bella English, "Boston Archdiocese Films AIDS Message," *Boston Globe*, March 26, 1987.

109 *"'But restraint does.'"*: Lisa Anderson, "Catholic Group's Anti-Condom Ads Draw Fire," *Chicago Tribune*, November 10, 1994.

110 *"he had visited 1,100"*: Charlie Rose interview with Cardinal John O'Connor, June 21, 1994.

10: "You Couldn't Say It Was Wrong"

114 *"Murder rates soared"*: Todd S. Purdum, "Murders Soar in 21 Precincts in New York," *New York Times*, March 24, 1987, https://tinyurl.com/hpj3msav.

117 *"which is how they met Will Wake"*: Author interview with Will Wake and James D'Eramo, September 20, 2018. Wake and D'Eramo are featured in a December 7, 2018, episode of the podcast *Nancy* titled "You Couldn't Say It Was Wrong," where an earlier version of the story was reported, available at https://tinyurl.com/yvsftfs6.

117 *"Will's partner, Jim D'Eramo"*: Lynda Richardson, "Proud, Official Partners," *New York Times*, August 1, 1993, https://tinyurl.com/3zuytscx.

11: Born This Way

124 *"wrote a letter to the editor"*: William Hart McNichols, "Cardinal Spellman and the Public," *New York Times*, November 25, 1984, https://tinyurl.com/n8zejxhn. Father McNichols was responding to a controversy over a book that claimed Cardinal Francis Spellman was a closeted gay man. Some argued the cardinal's sexual orientation was irrelevant since as a priest, he took a vow of celibacy. Bill disagreed, writing, "Cardinal Spellman's sex life does not matter, but Cardinal Spellman's homosexuality does indeed matter."

128 *"aversion therapy"*: Jamie Scott, "Shock the Gay Away: Secrets of Early Gay Aversion Therapy Revealed," HuffPost, June 28, 2013, https://tinyurl.com/y4trze4e.

130 *"a model of Christian forgiveness"*: Curtis Houlihan, "The Healing Touch: Father Bill McNichols and His Ministry to PWAs," *New York Native*, April 27, 1987.

12: Priests with AIDS

134 *"But he also had a pastoral side"*: Author interview with John Carr, September 25, 2020.

135 *"Tears filled his eyes"*: Author interview with Michael Sean Winters, October 5, 2020.

135 *"He spoke kindly of Father Mike"*: Doug Struck, "Hundreds at Cathedral Mourn Priest Dead of AIDS," *Baltimore Sun*, April 14, 1987.

135 *"responding to a reporter's question"*: "A Timeline of HIV/AIDS," AIDS.gov, https://tinyurl.com/9tmxvrpv.

136 *"to silence a gay Catholic organization in 1984"*: Jason Berry, "Homosexuality in Priesthood Said to Run High," *National Catholic Reporter*, February 27, 1987.

136 *"firm in our Catholic teaching"*: Mark Zimmerman, "Witnessing Priest's Death from AIDS 'Personalized' Illness, Archbishop Says," *Catholic Standard*, April 23, 1987.

139 *"in great disrepair"*: Stanley Ziemba, "CHA Seeks $12 Million to Upgrade Cabrini Homes," *Chicago Tribune*, January 30, 1975.

139 *"strong in spite of the challenges"*: Adam M. Rhodes, "A City within a City," *Chicago Reader*, March 30, 2021, https://tinyurl.com/y3hcp9fy.

140 *"God's special friends"*: Author interview with the Rev. Frank Latzko, February 12, 2021.

140 *"I'll bet 125 of those are Catholic":* Stephen Bryant, "Parish to Host Second AIDS Anointing Service," *Windy City Times,* October 1, 1987. Several of the quotes about Noone's early involvement with HIV and AIDS are taken from this article. The estimate that half of the city's 250 AIDS patients were Catholic in 1985 was likely very close to the mark; according to the archdiocese, 57 percent of the city's population was Catholic in 1970, and 48 percent in 2000. Archdiocese of Chicago, "Total Population Change in Archdiocese," *Data Composite: Facts and Figures for Year Ending 2019,* 9, https://www.archchicago.org/documents/70111/1884101/Data+Composite/4d71940f-8716-46aa-abd0-6dd6a35a6513.

142 *"had stymied progress":* Tom Gibbons, "Church Stand Seen as Key to Gay Rights Ordinance," *Chicago Sun-Times,* July 13, 1986.

143 *"homophobia could be crushing":* "AIDS: A Time for Healing," a report from the Archdiocese of Chicago AIDS Task Force, May 15, 1986.

144 *"had something important to say":* Author interview with Father Dominic Grassi, July 26, 2020.

146 *"his true cause of death":* "College Chaplain Succumbs to AIDS," United Press International, October 26, 1985.

146 *"until his death":* Bill Kenkelen, "AIDS Among the Clergy—a Public Test of Faith," *National Catholic Reporter,* January 4, 1987.

146 *"significantly higher than the general population":* See Miles Corwin, "Controversial Issue; Gay Priests: A Dilemma for Catholics," *Los Angeles Times,* February 16, 1987; and David Crumm, "Study Can't Figure Number of Gay Priests," *Detroit Free Press,* February 26, 1987. Richard Sipe, a former priest, is the source of the estimate. Sipe spent several decades writing about sexuality in the priesthood before his death in 2018. His work was featured in the 2015 film *Spotlight* about clergy sexual abuse.

146 *"as many as 26 percent":* Berry, "Homosexuality in Priesthood."

147 *"baloney":* Corwin, "Controversial Issue."

147 *"their fitness for the priesthood questioned":* Miles Corwin, "Priests with AIDS—'It's Important That People Know,'" *Los Angeles Times,* February 16, 1987, https://tinyurl.com/2fhmh3zw.

147 *"because of their illness":* Robert Lindsey, "AIDS among Clergy Presents Challenges to Catholic Church," *New York Times,* February 2, 1987, https://tinyurl.com/9t8tmwk9.

147 *"a problem that's affecting us":* Sandra G. Boodman, "Priests and AIDS: Will Church Minister to Its Own?," *Washington Post*, February 7, 1987.

147 *"Bishop Moore's insight":* Massa, "Vows of Silence." Bill McNichols also appears in this article, saying he hopes the church will see the courage of gay men of faith dying from AIDS.

148 *"Moore's death certificate":* Joe Sexton, "Death of a Bishop: Of Holy Orders and Human Frailty; Beloved Clergyman Hid Personal Battles," *New York Times*, October 7, 1995, https://tinyurl.com/6b8esbjy.

148 *"petitioned to have Moore's death certificate updated":* Pamela Schaeffer, "Breaking Silence: Priests with AIDS Are Eager to Talk," *National Catholic Reporter*, April 18, 1997, https://tinyurl.com/2t23xfzk.

148 *"HIV presented a challenge to their priests":* "Rev. Michael Peterson, Hospital Founder, Dies," *New York Times*, April 12, 1987, https://tinyurl.com/yxymsfew.

148 *"Father Mike Peterson's letter arrived":* Dan Chu, "As Father Michael Peterson Lay Dying of Aids, His Catholic Church Showed It Cared Deeply for One of Its Own," *People* magazine, May 11, 1987.

148 *"I have this lethal syndrome":* Jason Berry, *Lead Us Not into Temptation: Catholic Priests and the Sexual Abuse of Children* (New York: Doubleday, 1992), 254.

150 *"Father Jim's brother picked him up for Christmas dinner":* Author interview with Robert Noone, August 20, 2020.

151 *"unafraid of the truth":* Author interview with Michael Herman, May 15, 2020.

151 *"awed by his act of courage":* A few days later, a short obituary appeared on page nine of the *Chicago Tribune* and included: "Father Noone died at the parish rectory Wednesday from complications resulting from AIDS. He requested that it be mentioned in the sermon at his funeral." Kenan Heise, "James Noone, Pastor of St. Theresa," *Chicago Tribune*, February 1, 1991, https://tinyurl.com/2f3arpub.

13: Friends of Dorothy

154 *"They'd only give us their first name":* Elizabeth Fernandez, "Fear Bars the Door to a Haven," *San Francisco Examiner*, July 29. 1990.

154 *"That didn't sit well":* Author interviews with Michael Harank, October 18, 2020, and January 10, 2021.

155 *"solidarity with the poor":* Dorothy Day, "To Our Readers," *The Catholic Worker*, May 1933. Also see Tom Cornell, "A Brief Introduction to the Catholic Worker Movement," https://www.catholicworker.org/cornell-history.html.

156 *"the pages of this newspaper have been silent":* See John Loughery and Blythe Randolph, *Dorothy Day: Dissenting Voice of the American Century* (New York: Simon and Schuster, 2020), 361–62. This account of this episode is based also on author interviews with Michael Harank, January 12, 2021, and Carl Siciliano, March 5, 2020.

156 *"mentioned amongst you":* Dorothy Day, *The Duty of Delight: The Diaries of Dorothy Day*, edited by Robert Ellsberg (Milwaukee, WI: Marquette University Press, 2008), 551, 587.

156 *"Someone has to minister to gay people":* Rosalie Riegle Troester, *Voices from the Catholic Worker* (Philadelphia: Temple University Press, 1993).

156 *"his tactlessness":* Loughery and Randolph, *Dorothy Day*.

157 *"in her newspaper":* Webb, "Dorothy Day and the Early Years."

158 *"the crack cocaine crisis":* George Raine, "Cocaine Epidemic Threatens Medical Care for the Poor," *San Francisco Examiner*, January 5, 1989.

158 *"a single residential hospice":* "Bethany," undated newsletter from the Bethany Catholic Worker House.

158 *"an overwhelming sense of sadness and anger":* Harank, "Proposal to Establish."

159 *"peace and compassionate care":* "Bethany," undated newsletter.

159 *"Mother Teresa's hospice":* Sandra G. Boodman, "Neighbors Are Fearful of Nuns' Caring for the Dying in Convent," *Washington Post*, January 12, 1987.

160 *"You shouldn't be alone when you die":* Shuang Li, "Activist Nurse Michael Harank Remembers Oakland's Bethany House during AIDS Epidemic," *Oakland North*, December 7, 2018, https://tinyurl.com/s5wk4wau.

160 *"the spiritual writer Henri Nouwen":* Michael Ford, *Wounded Prophet: A Portrait of Henri J. M. Nouwen* (New York: Doubleday, 1999).

160 *"a priest who was gay":* John Murawski, "Henri Nouwen's intimate letters shed light on his 'theology of the heart,'" Religion News Service, October 5, 2016.

161 *"Pope Francis praised":* Pope Francis, "Visit to the Joint Session of the United States Congress," September 24, 2015, https://tinyurl.com/2k6tnjn8.

162 *"an upcoming Chicago election":* Maya Dukmasova, "Five Challengers Take on 46th Ward Alderman Cappleman from the Left," *The Chicago Reader*, February 18, 2019, https://tinyurl.com/38t9hpj2.

165 *"turned to friends":* "A Brief History of St. Catherine of Genoa Catholic Worker," from the Dorothy Day—Catholic Worker Collection, Raynor Memorial Libraries, Marquette University. Author interviews with James Cappleman, April 25, 2020, and Al Mascia, August 24, 2020.

168 *"demanding more respect for women and gays":* Jean Latz Griffin, "Gays, Women Look to Bernardin for Aid," *Chicago Tribune*, November 9, 1992.

168 *"This is us creating our own rituals":* Terry Wilson, "Gay Catholics Keep the Faith," *Chicago Tribune*, October 11, 1996, https://tinyurl.com/fa5r8bcm.

168 *"the house closed":* "A Brief History of St. Catherine of Genoa Catholic Worker."

169 *"objections of neighbors":* Daniel J. Lehmann and Suzy Schultz, "Catholics to Open AIDS residence," *Chicago Sun-Times*, September 3, 1987; and Tom Gibbons, "Should a Community Have the Right to a Voice in Whether a Home for AIDS Victims Locates in Its Midst?," *Chicago Sun-Times*, September 20, 1987.

169 *"consecrated their relationship":* Hal Dardick, "Chicago Alderman Going Out of State to Marry Partner," *Chicago Tribune*, October 10, 2013, https://tinyurl .com/7jwkx86k.

169 *"right to be ordained as a priest":* Nick Blumberg and Evan Garcia, "Neighborhood Issues May Fuel Uptown Race," WTTW, April 1, 2015, https://tinyurl .com/3mwumpyh.

14: A Tangible Love

172 *"I have no control over God":* Revson, "Mission to Heal."

173 *"a dizzying chorus of anguish":* Charles W. Bell, "AIDS Hits Gays in Religion; Raises Crisis of Ministering," *New York Daily News*, January 25, 1987.

174 *"He sobbed during the prayers":* Richard Pearson, "Ronald K. Bushnell, AIDS Activist," *Washington Post*, November 20, 1990.

174 *"the most Christ-like man I have ever met":* Brother Bert Ouellette, SC, "AIDS Ministry," *Church World*, June 28, 1990.

177 *"in the sanctuary today":* "Church of St. Francis Xavier Tour Guide," St. Francis Xavier, 2012, https://tinyurl.com/c2ysecxc.

15: REDEEMED IN SAN FRANCISCO

179 *"a few years ago"*: Author conversation with Archbishop John R. Quinn, November 19, 2016.

180 *"not having an abortion"*: This story is also recounted in John R. Quinn, "The AIDS Crisis: A Pastoral Response," *America*, June 28, 1986.

181 *"an accepting community"*: "The History of the Castro," KQED, https://www .kqed.org/w/hood/castro/castroHistory.html.

182 *"my guide for the afternoon"*: Author interview with Tom Battapaglia, November 6, 2019.

183 *"on the skids"*: Author interview with Father Tony McGuire, November 6, 2019.

184 *"rescinded the invitation"*: "Parish Rescinds Invitation to Gays," *Bay Area Reporter*, September 22, 1983.

184 *"end gay outreach"*: Paul Lorch, "Ed. Note," *Bay Area Reporter*, November 17, 1983. Lorch, the paper's editor, was responding to a letter from Father McGuire, in which McGuire canceled planned advertisements for Most Holy Redeemer in the paper, saying he disliked the pornography ads and that he found the paper's coverage of his decision to rescind the offer to host Dignity Masses "inaccurate and one-sided."

185 *"had disbanded an archdiocesan task force"*: Bill Kenkelen, "San Francisco Gays, Church at Standstill," *National Catholic Reporter*, July 15, 1983.

185 *"equating shacking up with marriage"*: Bill Kenkelen, "Quinn Attacks Measure on Gay 'Spousal' Rights," *National Catholic Reporter*, December 17, 1982.

187 *"I took the train to Oakland"*: Author interview with Cliff Morrison, November 5, 2019.

188 *"bridged the space between the gays and the grays"*: Donal Godfrey, *Gays and Grays: The Story of the Inclusion of the Gay Community at Most Holy Redeemer Catholic Parish in San Francisco* (Lanham, MD: Lexington Books, 2007), 80. Father Godfrey is a Jesuit priest who assists at Most Holy Redeemer and served as one of my tour guides during my visit to the parish in November 2019.

190 *"approached the parish"*: Charles Linebarger, "Hospice Proposed in Castro Convent," *Bay Area Reporter*, August 8, 1985.

190 *"supported the idea"*: "Former Convent Is San Francisco's First AIDS Hospice," UPI, March 3, 1987.

190 *"lively games of bingo":* "Bingo! Hospice Turns a Winner," *Bay Area Reporter*, May 8, 1986; and "Bingo Yields $10,000 for Coming Home Hospice," *Bay Area Reporter*, June 26, 1986.

191 *"We can't point the finger at anybody":* Don Lattin, "How AIDS Brought Gays and a Parish Together," *San Francisco Examiner*, July 28, 1986.

192 *"hundreds of people packed into Most Holy Redeemer":* Don Lattin, "Catholics Plan Prayer-a-Thon for AIDS Victims," *San Francisco Examiner*, August 22, 1985.

192 *"faulted Archbishop Quinn":* Ray O'Loughlin, "Archbishop Avoids Worst 2 Words," *Bay Area Reporter*, August 29, 1985.

192 *"wrote an essay":* Quinn, "AIDS Crisis."

192 *"A sign of his comfort":* Lattin, "How AIDS Brought."

193 *"still had not made a formal statement":* Robert Reinhold, "The Papal Visit: AIDS Issue at Fore as Pope Visits San Francisco," *New York Times*, September 17, 1987, https://tinyurl.com/49sxr259.

193 *"compassion in that direction":* Don Lattin, "The Diplomat," *Image*, August 30, 1987.

193 *"form an integrated parish":* Don Lattin, "Papal Visit to Hospice Is Urged," *San Francisco Examiner*, February 25, 1987.

194 *"Sister never batted an eyelash":* Godfrey, *Gays and Grays*, 42.

194 *"Despite that relative calm":* Lattin, "The Diplomat."

194 *"said was a photo op":* Elizabeth Fernandez, "Gays to Pope: Skip AIDS Hospice," *San Francisco Examiner*, April 15, 1987.

194 *"including two priests":* Associated Press, "2 Priests with AIDS Will Pray," September 9, 1987.

194 *"Demonstrators greeted the pope":* Associated Press, "Pontiff Draws First Big Protests of U.S. Tour," September 18, 1987.

194 *"objectively immoral behavior":* Associated Press, "Vatican Official Says AIDS Result of 'Immoral Behavior,'" September 10, 1987.

194 *"justice, mercy, and love":* Henry F. Rosenthal, "Pope Blesses AIDS Victims, Encounters Angriest Demonstrations," Associated Press, September 17, 1987, https://tinyurl.com/s43pnc3k.

195 *"ceased to be abstractions":* Lattin, "The Diplomat."

195 *"rectory at Most Holy Redeemer":* Author interview with Thomas Ellerby, November 6, 2019.

197 *"a parish that is full of love"*: Jane Meredith Adams, "The Castro 1988," *Boston Globe Magazine*, November 27, 1988.

197 *"the leading cause of death"*: Lawrence K. Altman, "AIDS Is Now the Leading Killer of Americans from 25 to 44," *New York Times*, January 31, 1995, https://tinyurl.com/5kf4j69d.

16: A Church Filled with Gospel Love

199 *"He didn't seek out the Polish pope"*: Stephen Martz, "Remembering Fr. Paul Murray," *Washington Blade*, February 13, 2009.

199 *"a crowd of 1,500 priests"*: Judith Valente and Patrick Tyler, "St. Matthews," *Washington Post*, October 7, 1979.

199 *"DC's gay newspaper"*: "Blade's 50 Year History Reflects Struggles, Advances of LGBT Community," *Washington Blade*, October 15, 2019, https://tinyurl.com/e6prv9t9.

201 *"lack of pastoral resources"*: Dominic E. Faraone, "Urban Rifts and Religious Reciprocity: Chicago and the Catholic Church, 1965–1996" (PhD diss., Marquette University, 2013).

201 *"church institutions didn't really have credibility"*: Author interview with Stephen Martz, January 15, 2021.

202 *"Steve stood up for other gay Catholics"*: Buursma, "Vatican Targets U.S."

204 *"Sex seemed to be everywhere"*: Author interviews with Guy Baldwin, January 25, 2021; Gary Chichester, April 30, 2020; and Dean Ogren, May 8, 2020.

205 *"a hunk who can talk"*: Lawrence Bommer, "Black Is Beautiful," *Windy City Times*, June 7, 1990.

205 *"more than half of Americans"*: Gallup, "Gay and Lesbian Rights," https://tinyurl.com/zvdj2hf3.

206 *"it even had its own AIDS ministry"*: Author interview with George Kuhlman, April 30, 2020.

206 *"one person out of every three hundred was diagnosed"*: Faraone, "Urban Rifts and Religious Reciprocity," 318.

208 *"looked in awe, and others with trepidation"*: Author interview with James Corrigan, February 18, 2021.

208 *"A group of drummers"*: Bommer, "Black Is Beautiful."

208 *"accepted for who they are"*: Author interview with Father Clete Kiley, May 4, 2020.

208 *"he got political"*: Lawrence Bommer, "Field of (Wet) Dreams," *Windy City Times*, June 1, 1989; and Bommer, "Black Is Beautiful."

210 *"a scene of quiet reverence"*: Faraone, "Urban Rifts and Religious Reciprocity," 329, 212.

211 *"to put God in that closet"*: Stephen Martz, "Case History: My Work with the AIDS Pastoral Care Network," 1985.

17: "Just Who the Hell Are These Two Nuns?"

215 *"akin to a leper colony"*: Oxford Biblical Studies Online, "Bethany," Oxford University Press, 2021, https://tinyurl.com/3mynev8h.

216 *"the GMHC version in New York"*: Mary Ellen Rombach, "AIDS Hotline," *Kinmundy Express*, February 9, 1989.

217 *"that woman"*: Roger Schlueter, "Bethany Place: Nuns Take on the World in Caring for People with AIDS," *Belleville News-Democrat*, October 21, 1991.

217 *"more people in Belleville living with HIV"*: Karisa Tavassoli, "AIDS in the Metro-East Area: The Politics of Treatment, Care, and Housing," Washington University St. Louis, February 3, 2017.

219 *"I'm Ted"*: The salon worker who was skeptical of Bethany Place but who eventually helped Carol and Mary Ellen raise funds is named Tom. His name was changed to Ted in this book for reader clarity. The name of George's partner in this chapter, whose name is rendered as Christopher, was also changed at the request of Carol.

219 *"she simply volunteered"*: Daniel R. Browning, "Counseling Service for AIDS Victims Gets Ultimatum," *St. Louis Post-Dispatch*, June 9, 1991.

220 *"great need for HIV education in Belleville"*: Cindy Humphreys, "Nuns Devote Lives to Helping AIDS Victims," *The Southern Illinoisan*, March 17, 1991.

221 *"understand the science"*: Chris Young, "A Call to Caring," *Heartland*, April 23, 1993.

221 *"look at your own biases"*: Roger Schlueter, "Love Helps Overcome AIDS Bias, Speakers Say," *Belleville News-Democrat*, November 7, 1992.

224 *"Whitney Houston at karaoke"*: Young, "A Call to Caring."

225 *"became activists themselves":* Associated Press, "City Sued over AIDS Shelter," June 15, 1989.

226 *"a Quonset hut":* Kevin McDermott, "Future of AIDS Shelter Looks Cloudy," *St. Louis Post-Dispatch*, December 12, 2004.

18: AIDS CRUCIFIXION

228 *"to chronicle in his books his friendships":* Daniel Berrigan, *To Dwell in Peace: An Autobiography* (San Francisco: Harper and Row, 1987).

230 *"support those with HIV and AIDS":* "Prayer Vigil Held," *Ram* (Fordham University), April 14, 1988, https://tinyurl.com/u8jp3tue.

231 *"red ink on beige paper":* William Hart McNichols, "Stations of the Cross of a Person with AIDS," 1989, https://tinyurl.com/aj98rncx.

232 *"tested positive for HIV":* Author interview with Stephen McDonnell, September 27, 2019.

235 *"aimed like an arrow":* William Hart McNichols, "For St Francis Day The Epiphany—Wisemen Bring Gifts to the Child," October 2017.

237 *"Inside the church's closet":* Amanda Ripley, "Inside the Church's Closet: Gay Priests Talk about Their Hidden Lives, Love of the Church and Fear of Being Scapegoated in the Sex Scandals," *Time*, May 20, 2002.

238 *"banned gay men from the priesthood":* Michael O'Loughlin, "Vatican Reaffirms Ban on Gay Priests," *America*, December 7, 2016, https://tinyurl.com/4pc6xtae.

238 *"Plague":* Plague is available at www.americamag.org/plague. Father McNichols is the subject of episode three, "The Cost of AIDS Ministry to a Gay Priest."

239 *"a 2005 interview":* Doug Cosgro, "Keeping the Faith," *Lavender*, December 9, 2005.

239 *"identified as a gay priest":* Michael J. O'Loughlin, "How the AIDS Epidemic Turned a Catholic Priest into an Art Activist," *Washington Post*, December 1, 2019, https://tinyurl.com/4stwky5a.

241 *"the patron saint of people with AIDS":* "Gonzaga: A Saint for AIDS Victims?," Catholic News Service, January 22, 1992.

241 *"make the association official":* "An Ancient Saint for a Modern Problem," *Catholic Herald*, January 31, 1992, https://tinyurl.com/4urm2nv9.

Epilogue

243 *"a feature on NPR"*: Phoebe Lett, "Podcasts about Beyoncé, Arias and Health Care: Worth a Listen," *New York Times*, December 8, 2019, https://tinyurl.com/xukbz4ue; Lulu Garcia Navarro, "How the Catholic Church Aided Both the Sick and the Sickness as HIV Spread," National Public Radio, December 1, 2019, https://tinyurl.com/468b7ve.

244 *"I'm being liberated"*: Author email exchange with Stephen Staten, December 27, 2019.

244 *"A sadness seems to accompany"*: For a look at the challenges facing long-term survivors of HIV, see the film Erin Brethauer and Tim Hussin, *Last Men Standing* (San Francisco: San Francisco Chronicle, 2016), documentary.

245 *"civil unions for same-sex couples"*: Michael J. O'Loughlin, "Pope Francis Declares Support for Same-Sex Civil Unions for the First Time as Pope," *America*, October 21, 2020, https://tinyurl.com/yv9cdwr6.

246 *"God 'does not and cannot bless sin'"*: "Responsum of the Congregation for the Doctrine of the Faith to a Dubium regarding the Blessing of the Unions of Persons of the Same Sex," The Vatican, March 15, 2021, https://tinyurl.com/tdfhdw27.

246 *"identify as Black"*: David Crary, "Black Catholics: Words Not Enough as Church Decries Racism," Associated Press, June 21, 2020, https://tinyurl.com/3sn2yk9c.

247 *"to take the epidemic more seriously"*: "Pastoral Plan of Action," National Black Catholic Congress IX, September 1, 2002, https://tinyurl.com/8crbw2k.

247 *"communities of color:"* "A Public Theology, Black and Catholic: HIV/AIDS in U.S. Communities of Color," by Bryan Massingale, delivered to the Black Catholic Theology Session of the Catholic Theological Society of America, June 10, 2000.

247 *"radically loved by God"*: Father Bryan Massingale, "The Challenge of Idolatry for LGBTI Ministry," a talk delivered to the Global Network of Rainbow Catholics, July 4, 2019, https://tinyurl.com/52dhstat.

249 *"a grueling pilgrimage in Spain"*: David Pais, "Making Camino de Santiago," *University of Notre Dame Alumni & Friends*, September 2, 2020.

Index